W9-DHL-455

ARTHRITIS

RELIEF

A TAKE-CHARGE PLAN
OF POSITIVE NUTRITION,
GENTLE EXERCISE,
RELAXATION,
MEDICAL CARE,
AND EVERYDAY COPING TIPS

by Jean Wallace, Ph.D.

Medical Advisers:
Bruce Hoffman, M.D., Medical College of Pennsylvania,
and
Jeffrey Lisse, M.D., University of Texas Medical Branch

 Rodale Press, Emmaus, Pennsylvania

Editor: Sharon Faelten

Research and Fact-Checking: Ann Gossy, Associate Research
Chief; Christine Dreisbach, Karen Feridun, Staci Hadeed, Dawn
Horvath, Karen Lombardi, Bernadette Sukley, Research Associates

Editorial/Production Coordinator: Jane Sherman

Copy Editor: Jill Caravan

Office Manager: Roberta Mulliner

Book Design: Denise Mirabello

Cover Design: Denise Mirabello

Illustrations: Stewart Jackson

Senior Managing Editor, Rodale Books: Carol Keough

Vice President and Editor in Chief, Rodale Books:
William Gottlieb

Senior Vice President and Managing Director, Rodale Books:
Pat Corpora

Group Vice President, Health: Mark Bricklin

Printed in the United States of America

If you have any questions or comments concerning this book,
please write:

> Rodale Press
> Book Reader Service
> 33 East Minor Street
> Emmaus, PA 18098

Library of Congress Cataloging-in-Publication Data

Wallace, Jean, Ph.D.
  Arthritis relief.

  Includes index.
  1. Arthritis—Popular works. I. Hoffman, Bruce, M.D. II.
Lisse, Jeffrey. III. Title.
RC933.W235 1989 616.7'22 89–6245
ISBN 0–87857–832–3 hardcover

Distributed in the book trade by St. Martin's Press

2 4 6 8 10 9 7 5 3   hardcover

Notice

The purpose of this book is to make the reader aware of progress in the management and treatment of common forms of arthritis. Proper diagnosis and treatment require expert advice. If you have arthritis, please seek competent medical help. The information here is designed to help you make informed decisions about your treatment. It is not intended as a substitute for any treatment prescribed by your doctor.

Contents

Acknowledgments

Many people contributed their time, expertise, and perspectives to the development of this book. Many thanks to them all, including Mary Brassell, R.N.; James M. Fox, M.D.; Victoria Gall, P.T., M.Ed.; Robert Gatter, M.D.; Diane Harlowe, M.S., O.T.R.; Charles L. Jones, D.P.M.; James R. Klinenberg, M.D.; Cynthia Stabenow Kulp, O.T.R.; Wendy McBrair, R.N.; Frederic C. McDuffie, M.D.; Earl C. Marmar, M.D.; Jodi Maron-Barth, P.T.; Janet R. Maurer, M.D.; Thomas C. Namey, M.D.; Evelyn Rossky, O.T.R./L.; Thomas P. Sculco, M.D.; Robert M. Stroud, M.D.; Stephen Wegener, Ph.D.; Michael E. Weinblatt, M.D.; and Beth Ziebell, Ph.D.

In addition, I am particularly indebted to Jeffrey Lisse, M.D., and Bruce Hoffman, M.D., for carefully reviewing the manuscript and suggesting changes. I also wish to acknowledge the Arthritis Foundation for providing a wealth of background information on rheumatic disease.

Special thanks, too, to my editor, Sharon Faelten; Carol Keough, William Gottlieb, Jane Sherman, Roberta Mulliner, Ann Gossy, Christine Dreisbach, Karen Feridun, Staci Hadeed, Dawn Horvath, Karen Lombardi, and Bernadette Sukley.

Finally, I am indebted to the many people with arthritis who shared their often inspiring stories in the hope of helping others. My thanks to: Howard MacDonald, Kathleen Kennedy, Jennifer DePalmer, Bill Warren, Linda Hoover, Betty Warner, Kathleen Lewis, R.N., Marie Stephenson, and Barbara Pollak.

Understanding
Arthritis

Take Charge
of Your Arthritis

Take this quick quiz and test your medical IQ.

1. What problem do actress Debbie Reynolds, baseball great Mickey Mantle, and world-renowned ballerina Suzanne Farrell have in common?

2. What is the most common chronic disease in people over age 45?

3. What medical condition can cost one person more than $150,000 in lost wages, medical care, and other expenses over a lifetime?

4. What potentially crippling disease can be controlled with gentle exercise, sound nutrition, rest, and a positive attitude?

The correct answer to all four is "arthritis." And by the time you finish reading this page, yet another American will receive a diagnosis of arthritis. Perhaps you're one of the million or so people struck by this disease each year—one every 33 seconds.

Statistics don't tell the whole story, though. Arthritis freezes joints that were formerly free and easy, making them stiff and painful. Movement becomes difficult, if not impossible.

Time was, all anyone could do for arthritis was to accept fate, learn to live with it, and take aspirin. But today, arthritis treatment is in the midst of a revolution. Newer drugs produce more complete relief, with fewer side effects. And surgeons can repair or replace creaky, worn-out joints.

Doctors are also looking beyond the pharmacy shelf and the operating room for ways to manage arthritis: They're helping people help themselves, by prescribing gentle exercise, recommending a change in diet, and encouraging them to adopt a positive attitude. Simply learning how to reduce emotional stress, for example, may help to keep arthritis in check. Studies show that people who believe in themselves, who have a can-do attitude, are more likely to overcome arthritis than people who give up.

"There's almost a direct relationship between how much responsibility people with arthritis take for themselves and how well they do," says Ted Pincus, M.D., a professor of medicine and microbiology at Vanderbilt University, Nashville, Tennessee. "If you take the approach that you can do something about your arthritis and solve this problem, then it's more likely your treatment will be effective."

Entertainer Debbie Reynolds, who has arthritis in her back and knees, says that exercise and a positive attitude have kept her going strong. She's been singing, dancing, and acting for years despite her often-painful condition. "I'm too stubborn to give up," she says. "I believe in taking care of myself because I don't want to have somebody else doing it for me. I can go and talk to a doctor, but he can't make me exercise. He can't make me do anything. *I* have to do it."

Like Reynolds, you, too, can lead a full and active life by developing your own personal plan for beating arthritis. Your two best allies are your doctor and the self-help strategies in this book. Your doctor can advise you on the best possible medical care for your particular situation, while this book will bring you up-to-date on the latest medical thinking about arthritis treatments and present dozens of medically approved self-help strategies that have worked well for others.

Distinguishing Facts from Fiction

Before you can begin to defeat arthritis, you need to know what you're up against. You can start by discarding common myths about the disease.

Myth #1: Arthritis is all the same.   Arthritis is not a single disease but a name for more than 100 painful conditions of the joints and associated connective tissues. Most are chronic, lasting a lifetime. Yet every case of arthritis is unique, and even people with the same condition can be affected differently—some suffer less pain than others, for example. The most common types are osteoarthritis and rheumatoid arthritis. (Various types of arthritis are explained fully in chapter 2, "The Many Faces of Arthritis.")

Myth #2: Nothing can be done for arthritis. You just have to learn to live with it.   That's pure hogwash. Just the opposite is true. Some types of arthritis can be completely controlled with medication. Although cures for most other types don't exist yet, you can do a great deal to reduce symptoms and live more comfortably. "There's really no person with arthritis who can't be helped in a substantial way," says James R. Klinenberg, M.D., a rheumatologist, professor of medicine at UCLA School of Medicine, and vice president of professional services at Cedars-Sinai Medical Center in Los Angeles. "Doctors can do a lot to manage arthritis and keep it under control."

Unfortunately, the notion that nothing can be done for arthritis keeps many people from seeking medical help. Take Hall of Fame baseball player Mickey Mantle, for instance. After retiring from baseball, Mantle developed arthritis in his knees. But he put off seeing a doctor because he assumed nothing could be done and that he was just getting old. An avid golfer, Mantle reached the point where he could hardly play the game anymore. Then, in 1987, he sought medical advice and underwent comprehensive medical treatment for his arthritis. Now he feels so much better that once again he plays golf several times a week. "I wish I'd known sooner what the right treatment could do for me," says Mantle.

Myth #3: Arthritis is an old person's disease. Arthritis commonly strikes people between the ages of 20 and 50, but it can affect folks of all ages, including infants and toddlers. The average person with arthritis is only 47 years old when it's first diagnosed, according to one survey. While it's true that osteoarthritis, the best-known form of the disease, becomes increasingly common as people grow older, many never develop any kind of arthritis at any time.

Myth #4: Exercise causes arthritis. Not long ago, doctors thought that if you used your joints too much, they would eventually wear out and develop arthritis. Now, everyone knows better. "Just as we recognize that exercise is good for the heart, we now know that exercise can keep the joints in good condition, too," says Warren A. Katz, M.D., chairman of the Department of Medicine and chief of rheumatology at Presbyterian/University of Pennsylvania Medical Center in Philadelphia. Studies have shown that people who exercise regularly, like long-distance runners, are no more likely to develop arthritis than anyone else. And for people who already have arthritis, gentle exercise does wonders for keeping joints healthy and flexible.

Perhaps this myth grew out of the fact that people who repeatedly abuse or injure their joints in sports or other physical activities *are* more prone to arthritis. "Exercise is good, but it has to be done in moderation," says Dr. Katz.

Myth #5: If you have arthritis, you'll eventually wind up crippled. "Only a very small percentage of people with arthritis become crippled," says Dr. Klinenberg. The vast majority never need a cane, wheelchair, or walker. If arthritis does progress to the point where you have difficulty walking, there's still hope. With joint replacement surgery—probably the single greatest medical advance for arthritis—many bad joints can be traded in for smoothly functioning artificial ones. These bionic parts can work so well that ballerina Suzanne Farrell kept on dancing with the New York City Ballet after receiving an artificial implant to replace her right hip, which osteoarthritis had worn away.

You may not be a prima ballerina, but your prospects for living a full and normal life despite arthritis are better than ever before. With the benefit of modern treatments and diagnostic tools, doctors can tell more quickly what kind of arthritis you have, then treat it more effectively. For most people, arthritis causes only mild or moderate symptoms, which, for the most part, can be relieved with good medical care and self-help strategies. "We're closer to finding a cure, and we have better drugs for management of arthritis than ever before," says Dr. Klinenberg. "We can better relieve the pain and suffering of patients. There are very good reasons to feel reassured and to feel positive that we can do something for you."

Spunk: Good Medicine for Arthritis

Determination. Courage. Optimism. Those traits, along with good medical care, are your best defense against arthritis. Take it from Bill Warren, who rode his bike 2,000 miles across the country, from Arizona to his boyhood town of Asheville, North Carolina, at age 66—despite arthritis. An artificial knee made the trek physically possible; a new outlook made it mentally possible.

Warren's left knee had become hopelessly damaged by osteoarthritis, which he developed as a young man. After surgery, he felt like a new man, free of pain for the first time in years. "On a scale of 1 to 10, I'd rate my improvement at about 400," he says. "It was just phenomenal."

While recovering from surgery, Warren began riding a stationary bicycle to strengthen his leg muscles. (Physical therapy helps an artificial joint to work properly.) He enjoyed cycling so much that he began to revive a long-forgotten dream of riding across country.

Warren had a few things going against him. One was his age. Also, he hadn't ridden a bicycle in years, and daily long-distance riding would require months of training. Even so, the surgeon who designed Warren's artificial knee was sure the stress of such rigorous cycling would destroy the implant. To top it off, Warren had a heart problem, and his cardiologist warned him against making the trip.

But Warren had powerful reasons for going ahead despite the odds. One was personal. His brother Fritz, who still lived in Asheville, had become depressed after having a stroke. In hopes of brightening his brother's outlook, Warren challenged him with a wager: If Warren would bike across the country to meet him, then his brother would make an effort to walk again. But Warren also wanted to share an important message with people in towns along his bike route. "I wanted to spread the message that there is an answer for people with arthritis other than 'learn to live with it,' " he says. "So many fine treatment options are available, joint replacement surgery being just one."

Riding about 50 miles a day, Warren completed his cross-country adventure in less than two months. When he arrived in Asheville, his artificial knee was working fine, and his heart was tremendously improved from the daily exercise. Like a triumphant Olympic contender, Warren was welcomed at the landmark Biltmore House estate in Asheville by his brother, family, friends, scores of jubilant well-wishers, and a crowd of news reporters.

Today, Warren is still active, riding his bike for short jaunts, playing golf, sailing, and walking his dog. During his cross-country trek, he gained many new insights into living with arthritis. He realizes that most people won't (or can't) cycle across the country, as he did. And most surgeons advise against such intense, grueling exercise for people with artificial joints. Still, he believes everyone with arthritis can benefit from setting goals for improving their lives, just as he did. "My goal was to ride 2,000 miles across the country," he says. "But to a grandmother with the same kind of pain I had, her one goal may be to walk around the yard leading her grandchild by the hand. That, too, is a worthwhile goal, and to achieve it is a monumental thing."

Whether your goal is to play golf, shed 15 pounds, or start a daily exercise routine, Warren believes it's important to work toward fulfilling your dreams by taking one small step at a time. "I didn't bicycle 2,000 miles. I bicycled 1 mile 2,000 times," he explains. "Unless you break your objective down into small increments, your goal may remain unreachable."

Perhaps the greatest wisdom Warren offers is that what counts the most is simply making an effort to improve your situation. "That's the real message for people with arthritis," he says. "If you don't try to do something for yourself, you're never going to accomplish a thing. You must try. You only fail when you don't try."

How This Book Can Help

The information in this book is not a substitute for medical advice. But it can help you to better understand your arthritis so you can make the best possible decisions about your treatments. You'll also find practical tips on everything from starting an exercise program to enjoying a more fulfilling love life.

Part 1, "Understanding Arthritis," explains the various kinds of arthritis and alerts you to symptoms that require prompt medical attention.

Part 2, "The Diet Connection," presents new findings about the controversial role of diet in causing or relieving arthritis symptoms. You'll also find a guide to help you distinguish well-founded dietary plans from harmful fad regimens.

Part 3, "Move Away from Pain," gives you step-by-step directions for embarking on various programs to exercise away pain and stiffness.

Part 4, "Using Your Mind and Emotions to Heal," tells you how to relax away pain, get a better night's sleep, and enjoy happier relationships. This section also offers strategies for coping with stress, fatigue, and depression—plus dozens of everyday coping tips.

Part 5, "Medical Help for Arthritis," explains what you need to know about arthritis drugs and surgery. Here you'll also find an objective look at alternative therapies to help you differentiate between helpful or harmless remedies and dangerous ones.

All in all, *Arthritis Relief* brings you the advice of dozens of physicians and other health care professionals in one handy reference guide. May it speed you toward recovery and relief.

2

The Many Faces
of Arthritis

Joints. Unseen and unheard, they bestow dexterity on pianists' deft fingers. They enable circus acrobats to somersault through the air and yoga devotees to contort themselves into human pretzels. They put the twist into Chubby Checker.

Without joints, your body might as well be frozen solid. You would be as immobile as the rusted Tin Man in *The Wizard of Oz* before Dorothy rescued him with an oilcan.

Although you rarely give your joints a second thought, they perform remarkable feats. Take your knee, for example. When you walk, the force transmitted through your knee is three or four times your total body weight. Squat down in a deep knee bend, and the force soars to nine times your weight. Even for a 100-pounder, that's hundreds of pounds of force pushing on the knees hundreds of thousands of times over a lifetime.

How do they do it? It's all in the design, as a quick tour of the inner workings of a joint shows. (See the illustration on page 10.)

A joint is formed at any place in the body where two bones meet. The ends of the bones are covered by a tough, elastic, compressible tissue called cartilage (or gristle) that keeps the bones from rubbing against each other.

The bones and cartilage of a joint are enclosed in a capsule. Tough and fibrous on the outside, the capsule is lined inside by a thin membrane called the synovium. Like Dorothy's oilcan, the

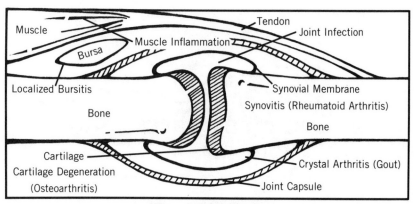

Muscle
Bursa
Muscle Inflammation
Tendon
Joint Infection
Localized Bursitis
Bone
Cartilage
Cartilage Degeneration
(Osteoarthritis)
Synovial Membrane
Synovitis (Rheumatoid Arthritis)
Bone
Crystal Arthritis (Gout)
Joint Capsule

Where Arthritis Attacks

synovium pours a lubricating fluid into the joint space, which reduces friction. So slippery is the joint fluid that when two bones are rubbed together, they create less friction than an ice skate gliding on a smooth frozen pond.

"If a jet engine's lubrication were as efficient as that of a pig's knee, it would be four times more efficient than it is now," states John H. Bland, M.D., rheumatologist at the University of Vermont College of Medicine in Burlington, in the *American Journal of Medicine*.

Cartilage and Muscle, the Joint Helpers

The cells that make up the cartilage are remarkable, too. Called chondrocytes, they are thought to live longer than any other cells in the body. Yet, nestled deep within cartilage, they are totally cut off from the life-giving nourishment of the blood supply. Instead, they draw their sustenance from the joint fluid.

Think of cartilage as a hard, fluid-filled sponge. During activity, the joint moves and the sponge is compressed. When you stop moving, the sponge expands, soaking up vital substances from the joint fluid.

This pumping action helps to keep the cartilage—and therefore the entire joint—healthy. Without a balance of rest and exercise, the chondrocytes (cells that make up the cartilage) cannot do their job, and the cartilage will fail. So, like your heart and lungs, joints require activity to remain healthy. It's a "use-it-or-lose-it" situation.

Muscles are the motors that drive the joints. They move the bones by contracting and relaxing. Muscles are attached to bones via strong, cordlike structures called tendons. Few people realize it, but muscles also act as shock absorbers, cushioning much of the impact of our movements. Ligaments, which are similar to tendons, connect bones and help to hold the joint together. Spread among the muscles and tendons are fluid-filled sacs called bursae that further cushion these moving parts.

Although you aren't aware of it, your brain, too, plays an important role in joint function. The brain is constantly communicating with the muscles via nerves, and this feedback is necessary for balance and to keep us prepared for our next movement.

Not convinced? "Consider what happens when we come down the stairs in the middle of the night to answer a ringing telephone, misjudge a step, and abruptly slip a couple of steps," say Kenneth D. Brandt, M.D., and Eric Radin, M.D., in an issue of *Hospital Practice.* "We feel a sharp jolt right up the spine—because our muscles are not prepared to accommodate the applied load."

Why Good Joints Go Bad

Unfortunately, joints don't come with a lifetime guarantee. Like other major organs, the joints and the soft tissues around them are vulnerable to an array of mishaps and maladies. Any part of a joint can become overstressed or affected by disease. The result? The stiffness, inflammation, and other symptoms that we know as arthritis.

More than 100 types of arthritis-related diseases exist, and the list of potential causes is mind-boggling. Germs, such as bacteria, can infect joints and cause arthritis. Injuries and overuse of a joint can lead in time to arthritis. Heredity, stress, viruses, drugs, and food allergies all have been implicated in some kinds of arthritis. But the fact is, no one really knows what causes most kinds of arthritis.

Mechanical malfunctions, too, can damage the joints. If the bones aren't lined up in the joint in just the right way, for example, the cartilage becomes stressed and wears out, causing osteoarthritis. For that reason, osteoarthritis is more common in people with skeletal alignment problems such as knock-knees or bowlegs. A good analogy is the extra wear on your tires when your car gets out of alignment. The abnormal distribution of pressure on the tires causes them to wear out faster than usual.

Finally, if your muscles are flabby, they perform like worn-out shock absorbers. They can't cushion the impact of movements, so the bones and cartilage absorb more shock than usual. Bones develop tiny fractures, and cartilage changes may in time lead to osteoarthritis.

Regardless of the cause, though, the end result of arthritis is often the same: stiff, painful, swollen, inflamed joints. And, unless you take steps to counter the problem, a vicious cycle can set in. As the joints become stiff, the muscles don't work as hard and they weaken through disuse. Weak muscles, in turn, increase the risk of injury to the joint and can aggravate arthritis.

The Role of Inflammation

Swollen, red, tender joints—the worst part of arthritis—are signs of inflammation, which is actually the body's natural way of protecting and repairing tissue that has been injured or affected by disease. The redness and heat result from blood rushing to joint tissues. Swelling occurs as white blood cells and fluid move into the tissues from the blood.

Inflammation works like a built-in burglar alarm system. If harmful bacteria, viruses, or any other foreign matter gets into the joint, the alarm goes off, bringing white blood cells, antibodies, and other body defense mechanisms to battle the intruders. Inflammation also is triggered when the joint is damaged by sports injuries or overuse.

But in some forms of arthritis, such as rheumatoid arthritis (RA), a dangerous false alarm seems to go off. Inflammation goes awry, turning on in a joint for no apparent reason. More seriously, the process refuses to turn off. If not kept in check, chronic inflammation can start to damage, rather than repair, joint tissues. In RA, this kind of inflammation has the potential, if unchecked, to destroy cartilage, bone, and ultimately the entire joint.

Osteoarthritis: The Democratic Disease

If you have osteoarthritis, join the crowd. This form of arthritis is probably the most common disease known to humankind. X rays can detect some signs of the disease in more than half the population by age 50. By age 70, the figure jumps to 85 percent.

Humans, by the way, are not suffering alone. Dolphins, whales, birds, hamsters, even your family cat or dog, get this kind of arthritis. The fossilized remains of a 200-million-year-old dinosaur show evidence of the disease. And some historians think that osteoarthritis of the spine was the reason cavemen walked with a stoop.

Ready to heave a huge sigh of despair? Save your breath. Although osteoarthritis is a nearly universal disease, it's not always painful or disabling. Compared to other forms of arthritis, it usually produces relatively mild symptoms. And in many people, the disease is silent. That is, while X rays may show some signs of osteoarthritis, the changes may not produce pain or discomfort for decades, if ever.

"The connection between the osteoarthritic changes that show up on an X ray and the pain and discomfort you actually feel is tenuous at best. There are thousands of people walking around with a substantial degree of osteoarthritis who feel no discomfort at all," says New York physician Willibald Nagler, M.D., in *Dr. Nagler's Body Maintenance and Repair Book.*

About 16 million people do have pain and discomfort from osteoarthritis, however. Women are twice as likely as men to develop this disease. Most often, symptoms begin after age 40, but osteoarthritis can strike earlier if your joints have been injured.

Osteoarthritis causes a deep, aching pain in one or more joints, especially those that bear weight, such as the hips, knees, and feet. The disease can also settle into the spine, where—surprisingly enough—it frequently causes no symptoms. Another form of osteoarthritis targets the hands, causing knobby enlargements of the finger joints and pain at the base of the thumb.

In osteoarthritis, the smooth cushions of cartilage at the ends of bones become pitted and frayed. In time, the cartilage may completely wear away, leaving the ends of bones unprotected. The bones also begin to grow and thicken in the joint, producing little bony spurs, or osteophytes, that can get in the way of normal movement and cause pain. Eventually, the joint begins to work like a rusted hinge rather than a well-oiled one.

Doctors used to think of osteoarthritis as a wear-and-tear disease. They assumed that, with age, cartilage inevitably wore thin, like the tread on a pair of tires after hundreds of miles of use. But modern researchers say it's unfair to blame age for osteoarthritis. Normal joints don't wear out with age, says Dr. Brandt, professor of medicine and head of the Rheumatology Division at the Indiana University School of Medicine. And, he says, the joint changes in normal aging are different from the joint changes in osteoarthritis. "It's possible that aging and osteoarthritis are two absolutely independent things."

So what does cause osteoarthritis? It may be that an insult to the joints when we're young sets off a gradual process that causes symptoms to appear years later. Or years of repeated out-of-the-ordinary demands on a joint may eventually lead to osteoarthritis. Osteoarthritis is more common in the toes of ballet dancers, for example, presumably because they spend so much time standing and landing on their toes. Similarly, basketball players tend to develop osteoarthritis in their knees, while miners get it in the spine, probably from lifting and shoveling heavy loads.

"The development of osteoarthritis can often be traced to abnormal or increased stress to a joint," writes Dr. Bland in *Running and Fit News,* the newsletter of the American Running and Fitness Association. "That is, when a joint is continually stressed in a way that it was not meant to be stressed, it can become injured, and possibly osteoarthritis can develop." People who are overweight are also more likely to develop osteoarthritis, studies show.

As later chapters will explain more fully, a careful exercise program to keep joints flexible and muscles strong is one important way to both prevent and treat osteoarthritis. Shedding excess pounds also can reduce stress on joints and relieve pain. Aspirin is widely used to relieve symptoms. Some people use canes or self-help devices to protect their damaged joints. In severe cases, surgery to replace worn joints with artificial ones can relieve pain and restore function.

Rheumatoid Arthritis: The Whole-Body Illness

Into each life a little pain must fall. But for people with RA, the pain is unpredictable and as a result can play on the emotions. You can be elated on a day when you feel almost back to normal, then grimly depressed when the pain returns full force.

In the early stages of the disease, joints in the hands and feet often become swollen, warm, and painful. Other main targets are the elbows, cervical spine, and (later) the knees. Joint pain tends to be symmetrical, meaning the same joint hurts on each side of the body. RA is often called a morning disease because many people feel stiff after they wake up—another early symptom.

Unlike osteoarthritis, RA may affect other parts of the body. Someone with RA may experience fever, loss of appetite, and a general "washed-out" feeling. Anemia (too few red blood cells), inflammation of the eyes, and pleurisy, which makes breathing painful, may also develop. Sometimes lumps called rheumatoid nodules appear under the skin, especially at the backs of the elbows. The lumps tend to come and go and usually don't cause problems other than cosmetic ones.

Still, RA is one of the most serious forms of arthritis, with the potential to cause deformity and crippling. Luckily, only a small number of people affected—about one in six—will develop deformed joints, according to the Arthritis Foundation.

"There are many people who just have mild disease," says Karin V. Straaton, M.D., a rheumatologist and assistant professor of medicine at the University of Alabama in Birmingham. "Especially with good medical care, many people do lead normal lives."

How to Prevent Osteoarthritis

Chances are you already know you can help to prevent heart disease by not smoking, watching your cholesterol, and getting regular exercise. But did you know that many of those same sound health habits are important for lowering your risk of arthritis, too?

Doctors say they don't know enough about what causes arthritis to be able to tell people how to prevent all of its various forms. But many believe you can take steps to reduce your risk of osteoarthritis, the most common type of arthritis.

What's more, it's never too late to begin "arthritis-proofing" your joints. Even if you already have arthritis, you can still benefit from building a strong musculoskeletal system. Many of these tips also can help to reduce the pain and discomfort of osteoarthritis, if you have it.

A joint-healthy lifestyle includes these habits.

Getting fit. Exercise is essential for healthy cartilage, and it strengthens the muscles, tendons, and ligaments that keep joints working properly. Exercise keeps the bones strong, too, by preventing calcium loss. "In general, the recommendation for a person who is well, who is not having joint pain, would be to remain active, to maintain muscle tone and range of motion," says Kenneth D. Brandt, M.D., of the Indiana University School of Medicine.

Paying attention to pain. Pain is the body's way of telling you to ease up before it's too late. If pain bothers you, cut back a little or change temporarily to a less stressful activity, such as swimming. "With

About two million Americans have RA, and three-quarters of them are women. The disease usually affects women during their childbearing years, but children and the elderly can get it, too.

Occasionally, symptoms of RA show up with no warning whatsoever. More often, though, the disease comes on slowly, and neither the person nor the doctor may know at first what's wrong. It can then continue to flare up—or it may disappear on its own as mysteriously as it arrived. In one out of five people affected, it disappears for good.

The basis for rheumatoid arthritis is chronic inflammation in the synovium, or joint lining. The normally thin membrane begins exercise, you may feel some muscle soreness, but it should disappear very quickly," says James M. Fox, M.D., medical director of the Center for Disorders of the Knee in Van Nuys, California. Pain that persists "is a sign that we're overdoing things or that there's something mechanically wrong in the joint."

Have you seen or heard the slogan "no pain, no gain" in gyms? Well, ignore it. Dr. Fox says it ought to be amended to read: "No pain, no gain, no brain!"

Being kind to your joints.   If you have an old injury in a joint, ease up on pounding exercises such as jumping rope or jogging. Do the same if you have a joint alignment problem such as knock-knees or bow-legs. (An operation called an osteotomy may be able to fix a malaligned joint; ask your doctor.)

Cushioning your feet from shock.   Minimize stress on your joints by wearing shock-absorbent shoes, such as those with heavily cushioned soles. Also. wear shoes that fit well and that are specially designed for the activity. A resilient surface, such as ground or a wood floor, also puts less stress on joints than hard concrete.

Keeping your weight down.   Recent studies show that people who are overweight are more likely to develop osteoarthritis. Also, people who are overweight are more apt to be sedentary and forgo the activity needed for healthy joints. (For weight-loss tips, see chapter 4, "Anatomy of a Healing Diet.")

to swell and thicken in the areas around the cartilage and bone. This tissue, called a pannus, can release destructive substances that eat away at joint tissues. In other words, the immune system runs amok, attacking the very tissues that it's designed to protect. Why that happens, no one knows. Some scientists believe heredity may play a role in RA, perhaps by making a person more susceptible to the illness.

Stress also seems to be instrumental in RA, if not in causing the disease then certainly in making it worse. One woman, for example, developed symptoms three days after her son committed suicide. Another felt joint pain for the first time after seeing her husband return from the operating room after having a brain tumor removed. "Stress certainly seems to be a factor, but its mechanism remains a mystery," says Warren A. Katz, M.D., a Philadelphia rheumatologist, in his book *Rheumatic Diseases: Diagnosis and Management.*

Although no cure exists for RA, much can be done to relieve pain and prevent damage to the joints. As later chapters will explain, exercise and physical therapy are important. Drugs to reduce inflammation, such as aspirin in high doses, are widely used. More powerful drugs can put the disease into remission. Increasingly, surgery to replace damaged joints helps many people.

Juvenile Rheumatoid Arthritis

Scrapes. Cuts. Bruises. Most kids' bodies take the battering that comes with learning to skate or ride a two-wheeler. Other kids experience much more pain—without ever skating or biking. They have an illness known as juvenile RA.

Although it shares the same name as the RA of adults, that's where the similarity ends. For one thing, juvenile RA is not one disease but an umbrella term for several related illnesses. In all, about 71,000 children nationwide have juvenile RA.

The general definition of juvenile RA is straightforward: persistent arthritis that lasts at least six weeks in any child under 17. Beyond that, there are three main types. The first, called systemic-onset, begins dramatically with a high fever and causes an array of whole-body symptoms in addition to arthritis. The second type affects only a few joints and is called pauciarticular. (*Pauci* means few and *articular* means joints.) The third type affects mostly girls who have arthritis in many joints. It is called polyarticular, because *poly* means "many."

The outlook for most kids with juvenile RA is surprisingly bright. About 80 percent will fully recover, with no permanent disabilities, says Ilona S. Szer, M.D., an assistant professor of pediatrics at Tufts University School of Medicine and associate director of the Division of Pediatric Rheumatology at the Floating Hospital for Infants and Children, both in Boston.

The goal of treatment is to allow children to remain active and live as normally as possible, says Dr. Szer. Besides taking high doses of aspirin to relieve joint inflammation, children need daily physical therapy to keep their muscles strong and their joints flexible. That way, if and when the disease eventually burns itself out, the children will still have healthy musculoskeletal systems.

"We tell kids they can do anything," says Dr. Szer. "If they want to play football, we tell them 'that's fine, but you have to do your physical therapy first.'

"We don't cure this disease," she adds. "We wait for it to go away, and in the majority of patients, it does go away."

Gout: The Arthritis of Kings

Gout sneaks up on an otherwise healthy person with no warning. Typically, the ambush occurs in the big toe, which suddenly turns hot, swollen, and dusky red with inflammation. The pain is so intense it wakes you from a sound sleep. It is so terribly exquisite, the surprised victim may be unable to bear even the weight of a sheet. It is so severe that the slightest jarring of the bed sets off shock waves of agony.

No wonder that gout once was called *podagra,* from the Greek term for seizure of the foot. "There's nothing subtle about a gout attack," says Bruce Hoffman, M.D., chief of rheumatology at the Medical College of Pennsylvania in Philadelphia. "It's a memorable experience—and an extremely painful one."

Fortunately, if gout does declare war on you, you can fight back and win. You can prevent future attacks by taking medications and keeping a watchful eye on your eating and drinking habits. "If you have gout, you can expect that, if you follow the correct regimen, you will be completely normal," says Frederic C. McDuffie, M.D., formerly senior vice president of medical affairs for the Arthritis Foundation and now director of the arthritis unit at Piedmont Hospital, both in Atlanta.

About one million Americans have gout, mostly men who develop the disease between the ages of 30 and 50. Women, who are protected from the disease thanks to differences in the kinds and amounts of sex hormones released by their bodies, seldom get gout until after menopause.

A gout attack, even if untreated, will go away by itself in anywhere from a few hours to several weeks. But without proper care, the disease can resurface and stage more menacing and frequent attacks. If unchecked, gout can spread to other joints, causing permanent damage. It also can damage the kidneys and cause hard lumps called tophi to form under the skin.

The cause of all this grief is well established. A gout attack occurs when crystals of uric acid, a natural body chemical, find their way into the joint. Like tiny needles or shards of glass, these microscopic crystals set off the stabbing pain and inflammation of gout. Besides attacking the toe, gout can inflame ankles, insteps of the feet, knees, elbows, wrists, and fingers.

Uric acid is a waste product formed from the breakdown of other substances called purines. Normally, uric acid does not form crystals. Rather, it dissolves in the blood and other body fluids. All people with gout have too much uric acid in their tissues. Some people also have too much uric acid in their blood, a condition called hyperuricemia. In both groups, gout attacks occur when the excess uric acid in the tissues forms crystals.

Most people with gout have a kidney problem that prevents them from getting rid of uric acid fast enough. Others may produce too much uric acid. Eating or drinking foods that are high in purines also can raise uric acid levels and trigger gout.

Mysteriously, most people with high uric acid levels never develop gout. In others, the uric acid level may be excessive for years before gout occurs. That's why a doctor should never say you have gout based only on a blood test for uric acid, says Dr. Hoffman. Rather, your physician should see if crystals are present in a sample of joint fluid or one of the nodules. (See chapter 3, "When to See Your Doctor.")

If you have gout, your doctor will probably recommend medications to lower your blood uric acid. Should another attack of gout begin in any joint, taking an anti-inflammatory drug at the first sign of trouble will stop the pain and inflammation.

A few simple dietary changes can maximize relief from gout. The Arthritis Foundation suggests:

• Drink alcohol in moderation, if at all. Many alcoholic beverages are high in purines, which can raise uric acid levels into the danger zone.

- Avoid crash dieting. Very-low-calorie diets can temporarily raise uric acid levels and aggravate gout.
- Eat certain rich foods sparingly. Liver, brain, fish roe, kidney, mussels, and anchovies are high in purines and should be eaten only occasionally, if at all.

Arthritis That Isn't: Tendinitis and Bursitis

Sometimes an ache that feels like arthritis isn't. That is, the pain comes not from inside the joint but from the surrounding soft tissues—the muscles, ligaments, and tendons. If the pain comes from inflammation of a tendon, it's called tendinitis. If it comes from a bursa, it's called—you guessed it—bursitis.

Overdoing any kind of physical activity is the usual cause of soft-tissue problems. Tennis elbow, for example, is so common that about half of the 35 million tennis players nationwide will develop it at some point, estimates one physician. Tennis elbow is a form of tendinitis that occurs when one of the tendons that attach forearm muscles to the elbow becomes inflamed.

But you don't have to be a fitness buff to sustain soft-tissue injuries. Any kind of overuse will do it. Just ask a video-game player with a case of Pac-Man thumb, caused by stress to the thumb from playing the game. Or a gambler with slot-machine tendinitis, a sore shoulder from trying too doggedly for the jackpot. Not to mention those who've had housemaid's knees, a form of bursitis resulting from too much kneeling, or shopping bag syndrome, a painful shoulder from lugging a heavy bag.

Soft-tissue rheumatism is one of the most common causes of musculoskeletal pain—and one of the most readily treated, doctors say.

Unlike the persistent pain of arthritis, soft-tissue problems usually heal on their own in a few weeks. Ease up on whatever activity caused the pain for as long as you feel sore. Rest your tender joint and apply a bag of ice for 10 to 15 minutes every 2 hours for two days or until the swelling subsides. (See your doctor if pain and swelling last longer than two days.)

Fibromyalgia: The "Princess and the Pea" Syndrome

Are you a perfectionist reporting to a workaholic? Settling a lawsuit out of court while negotiating your divorce? Expecting twins, buying a house, and starting your own business? If your daily life seems like an endurance test, you may be a candidate for fibromyalgia, a common musculoskeletal ailment that often targets overstressed people.

Fibromyalgia (also called fibrositis) is another example of soft-tissue rheumatism. People with fibromyalgia have chronic, widespread, unexplained pain in the muscles and other soft tissues around the joints, often with sleep and mood disturbances. Although the joints may feel stiff or swollen, they are not affected.

Fibromyalgia affects far more women than men. Although it is never a life-threatening illness, people who have it often feel tired and depressed. Typically, their aches become worse with stress or cold, wet weather, and better with a relaxing vacation (although stress does not cause fibromyalgia in every case). People with fibromyalgia tend to sleep poorly—an important clue to the cause of this mysterious malady.

"It may be that whatever disturbs our sleep can lead to the symptoms of fibromyalgia," says P. Kahler Hench, M.D., a fibromyalgia researcher and a senior consultant in the Division of Rheumatology at the Scripps Clinic and Research Foundation in La Jolla, California.

What does sleep have to do with how our bodies feel? A great deal, Dr. Hench says. If the normal deep stages of sleep are disturbed, the brain—the organ that registers pain—begins to overreact to normal sensations from soft tissues. Like the princess in the fairy tale who couldn't sleep when a tiny pea was placed under her mattress, people with fibromyalgia are unusually sensitive to even minimally painful stimuli.

Experienced doctors can predict just where they will find tender spots—called tender points—in people with fibromyalgia. Researchers are still trying to determine if there is anything wrong with the seemingly normal tissues there. The problem may also rest partly in how the brain reacts to the pain, Dr. Hench says.

Many people may develop fibromyalgia because stress disrupts their sleep, he says. Fibromyalgia also can occur with other illnesses, perhaps because pain or discomfort interferes with sleep.

"It's a combination of physical and emotional stress," agrees Richard T. Swanson, M.D., a clinical associate professor of medicine at the University of Indiana School of Medicine and head of the rehabilitation center and rehabilitation services at Welborn Hospital in Evansville. "It's commonly seen in people who stop taking care of themselves."

Conversely, doctors know that physically fit people are less likely to develop the ailment, and exercise helps to protect against it. Thus, treatments often include the following strategies.

Simple reassurance. People with fibromyalgia need to know that they don't have a more serious underlying condition.

Better sleep. Simple changes in sleep habits may help. (See chapter 10, "The Three Rs: Relaxation, Rest, and Relief.") Some doctors also prescribe medications such as Elavil or other tricyclic antidepressants to promote better sleep. These medicines are not the same as sleeping pills. Sleeping pills are not the best solution because they do not provide full and natural sleep.

Exercise. "Most people will tell you that with a little exercise they feel better and they sleep better," says Dr. Hench.

Learning to relax and manage stress. Whether it's by soaking in a bubble bath or teeing off at the golf course, you need to make some time for yourself every week, says Dr. Swanson.

Ankylosing Spondylitis: The Ultimate Stiff Back

True, it has an odd jawbreaker of a name, but ankylosing spondylitis is an all-too-common cause of pain and stiffness in the back, particularly in young men.

Actually, the name says it all, once you know how to decode it: The words mean stiffness (*ankylosis*) of the vertebrae (*spondylos*) with inflammation (*itis*).

And that's just what happens. For unknown reasons, chronic inflammation occurs where the tendons and ligaments connect the vertebrae in the spine. Over several years, the disease runs its course and the inflammation subsides. But in the process of healing, the normally flexible vertebrae may fuse together into a single stiff column, sometimes called a poker spine.

About 318,000 Americans, mostly men, have some signs of ankylosing spondylitis. Women develop the disease, too, but usually in a milder form. Pain in the lower back and legs is the most common symptom of the disease, which is somewhat hereditary. (This is not to be confused, however, with the kind of low back pain and morning stiffness that are associated with mechanical problems and are usually relieved by activity.) Some people also feel tired, lose their appetite, or run a fever.

While there is no cure for ankylosing spondylitis, anti-inflammatory drugs such as indomethacin can help. Self-care measures are equally important. The Ankylosing Spondylitis Association, a national self-help organization based in Los Angeles, offers these tips.

Stand tall. By vigilantly practicing good posture, people with ankylosing spondylitis can avoid being permanently stooped over if their spines do fuse. (To remind yourself what constitutes good posture, stand with your back against the wall.)

Exercise. It's important to keep the back flexible and relieve pain. (Swimming is especially good.)

Avoid soft, fluffy chairs. Hard chairs help to keep the spine straight.

Sleep on a firm mattress. A firm bed is another way to keep the spine straight, as is sleeping without a pillow—or with just a small one.

Lupus: A War Within

The name alone is frightening: systemic lupus erythematosus, or lupus for short. Named after the Latin word for wolf, lupus can be as unpredictable as its namesake. (Lupus got its name because in the 1880s, common lupus—another form that's caused by a form of tuberculosis that affects the skin— left people looking like they'd been bitten on the face by a wolf. The name stuck.)

About 131,000 Americans, mostly women and many blacks, contract this multisymptom disease. Lupus typically begins between the ages of 20 and 40, but it can strike anytime.

Most people with lupus have arthritis. The joint problems, however, are relatively mild, and it is the disease's potential harm to the other organs—the heart, lungs, kidneys, and brain—that make lupus a potentially life-threatening illness.

The early symptoms are variable. Besides arthritis, most people with lupus have fever and feel tired. About half have chest pains, caused by inflammation of the tissues that line the heart and lungs. Some people develop a rash in the shape of a butterfly across their nose and cheeks, which worsens in the sun.

Although it can be fatal, the disease is far from life-threatening in most cases. And, as with RA, the symptoms of lupus can come and go, suddenly disappearing for good in some people.

Unfortunately, doctors have not yet found a way to stop lupus. But much can be done to tame the illness and hold its symptoms at bay. "Today, the likelihood of a lupus patient's living at least a decade is over 90 percent and rising; probably most can look forward to a normal or near-normal life span," writes Sheldon P. Blau, M.D., in his book *Lupus: The Body against Itself.*

The cause of lupus has baffled scientists for more than a century. The list of potential culprits—viruses, environmental chemicals, heredity—is long enough to perplex Sherlock Holmes. Like RA, lupus is an autoimmune disease, in which the normally benevolent immune system attacks the body. Treatment is aimed at reducing inflammation and, in some cases, suppressing the immune system.

Lyme Disease:
Arthritis from a Bug Bite

What could be more fun than a bracing tramp through the woods? But if you live in some parts of the country, beware: A healthful outing could lead to an insidious form of arthritis called Lyme disease, transmitted by tick bites.

Virtually unknown 25 years ago, this ailment is now the most common tickborne disorder in the United States.

Lyme disease is named after the town in southern Connecticut where it was first identified in 1975. The illness was reported in 43 states in 1988 and is especially prevalent in the Northeast (in coastal areas), the northern Middle West (Minnesota and Wisconsin), and the West.

"Anyone who lives in or visits an area where Lyme disease is endemic is susceptible to the condition," say researchers from the State University of New York at Stony Brook in *Scientific American.* "Lyme disease is indiscriminate; it affects both sexes and all age groups."

The pinhead-sized ticks responsible for Lyme disease carry a harmful microbe called a spirochete, which actually causes the illness. The ailment usually begins like the flu, causing chills, fever, fatigue, and muscle and joint aches. A red bump that expands into a rash usually appears at the site of the tick bite. If untreated, Lyme disease can resurface in weeks or months in new guises. Some people experience heart palpitations, chest pains, shortness of breath, and nervous system problems. Months later, in its final stages, Lyme disease can attack the joints and cause chronic arthritis.

At any stage, antibiotics can stop the disease cold. But Lyme disease is not always easy to diagnose. To be certain, doctors can use a blood test that detects antibodies, or protective substances in the blood, to the microbe.

If you live in an area where Lyme disease is common, do whatever you can to avoid tick bites, especially when the ticks are most active—from late spring to early fall. Here's how.

• When outdoors, wear a hat and protective clothing that keeps you covered. Tuck long pants into your socks or boots.
• When you return home, check your whole body carefully, including your scalp. Remember, you're looking for a speck-sized tick that might pass for a tiny mole.
• If you find a tick, gently grasp it with fine-tipped tweezers and pull it straight up and out. Ticks are tiny, so be careful not to crush the tick or leave its head embedded in your skin. Also,

never touch a tick with your bare hands. Save the tick in a small jar of alcohol; it may help your doctor with a diagnosis should you develop symptoms of Lyme disease.

Other Types of Arthritis

The types of arthritis described so far account for well over 80 percent of all cases. There are other, less-common types.

Infectious arthritis. The same bacteria that can cause gonorrhea, tuberculosis, and meningitis sometimes infect the joints, leaving them hot, red, painful, and swollen. Joint infections can be cured with antibiotics, but prompt treatment is crucial to prevent joint damage.

Reiter's syndrome. Reiter's syndrome, which occurs mostly in men, causes a variety of symptoms besides arthritis. It usually is associated with pinkeye, or inflammation of the eye, a red rash on the genitals or feet, and discharge from the urethra.

Psoriatic arthritis. Many people have psoriasis, a chronic skin problem that causes red, scaly patches on the body. A small number, about 5 percent, also develop a form of arthritis that is directly related to psoriasis. In many people, the symptoms are mild and may require no treatment.

Scleroderma. Scleroderma, which means "hard skin," causes the skin on the face and hands to become stiff and tight, with a leathery texture. Besides damaging the extremities, it can harm internal organs, including the esophagus, heart, lungs, and kidneys. Scleroderma is rare, and no one knows what causes it.

Polymyalgia rheumatica. This disease causes muscle aches in older people, mainly in the muscles of the neck, shoulder, lower back, hips, and thighs. Most people get better quickly after treatment, which usually consists of low doses of corticosteroids.

So, there you have it—13 of the most common forms of arthritis, and a starter kit of information on how to manage the pain, swelling, and stiffness they can cause. For more information on what you can do to tame the more common and stubborn forms of this ailment, read on.

Warning Signs of Arthritis

How, when, and where you ache may indicate which kind of arthritis you're experiencing.

Osteoarthritis

- Mild aching or soreness, especially when moving joints.
- For some, symptoms may get worse with activity and better with rest. Others may have nagging pain, even at rest.
- Joints may be stiff and hard to move.

Rheumatoid Arthritis

- Pain and stiffness in joints, followed by tenderness and swelling. The same joint on each side of the body is usually affected.
- Stiffness, fatigue, and aching in the morning or after long rests.
- Loss of appetite, fever, or weight loss.

Juvenile Rheumatoid Arthritis

- Joint pain and swelling.
- Child may be stiff and sluggish in the morning or after naps.
- Sometimes a high fever, a rash, or other whole-body symptoms precede joint pains.

Gout

- Sudden onset of an intensely painful joint, along with swelling, redness, and heat. Often occurs first in the big toe.
- Skin over affected joint may appear red or purple and shiny.
- Joint may be tender to even the slightest touch.

Fibromyalgia

- Generalized aches and stiffness that persist for three months or longer.

- Symptoms may worsen in damp, cold weather or with stress.
- Possibly tiredness, anxiety, sleep disturbances, and depression.

Ankylosing Spondylitis

- Pain in the lower back and legs that develops gradually, usually within weeks rather than hours.
- Early morning stiffness and pain.
- Exercise relieves symptoms and rest worsens them.
- Symptoms persist for more than three months rather than occurring in sporadic attacks.

Lupus

- Fatigue, fever, depression, and joint pains.
- Often hair loss and rashes that worsen upon exposure to sunlight.
- Fingers may become blue and white when exposed to cold.
- Assorted other symptoms affecting major organs.

Lyme Disease

- Usually characterized by a distinctive rash consisting of a bump surrounded by a gradually spreading red zone.
- Flulike symptoms, with fever, chills, malaise.
- In time, arthritis, heart palpitations, or nervous system disorders.

If you have arthritis, chapter 3, "When to See Your Doctor," will help you get the medical guidance needed to diagnose and manage its symptoms.

CHAPTER
3

When to See Your Doctor

In one survey, about 30 percent of people who developed arthritis waited a year before seeing a doctor, and 15 percent waited more than two years. But procrastination is a *mistake.*

"Early diagnosis is crucial so the appropriate treatment can begin before the joints are irreversibly damaged," says Colin J. Dunn, Ph.D., an arthritis researcher with the Upjohn Company, which conducted the survey.

Peace of mind is another benefit of going to the doctor right away. "The most important reason to see your doctor is to find out about your symptoms," says Frederic C. McDuffie, M.D., former senior vice president of medical affairs for the Arthritis Foundation. "Is this something that's serious, that's going to affect your life? Your family? Your job?"

According to the Upjohn report, most people put off seeing their doctor because their symptoms don't seem severe or persistent—they just don't think they have arthritis. Others blame a recent strain or injury for their discomfort.

The world's record for putting off that first doctor's visit goes to a woman who waited *30 years* to see a doctor about her rheumatoid arthritis (RA). "She didn't think anything could be done for her," says Michael E. Weinblatt, M.D., a Boston rheumatologist who treated the woman when she finally did seek help. "She came into the clinic in a wheelchair. She hadn't been able to walk in ten years." The woman's joints were so badly damaged that she needed seven joint replacement operations: two hips, two knees, two shoulders, and an elbow. She's walking again, but if she had sought help earlier, such drastic surgery might not have been necessary.

While this woman's case shows the folly of waiting to seek treatment, it also tells us that it's *never* too late to get help. The course of many arthritis-related diseases is slow, and damage to the joints usually happens gradually. Even if joint damage has occurred, surgery may be able to correct deformities or replace joints. And in most cases, all you'll need is medication and counseling on how to cope with the condition.

The Signs of Severity

Most minor musculoskeletal problems heal on their own within two to six weeks, says James Fries, M.D., in the *Textbook of Rheumatology*. But joint pain that lasts longer than six weeks is a cue to seek medical attention. And if other symptoms are present, see your doctor sooner.

"If the movement of the joint is very much limited, if there's redness or swelling with pain in a joint, you should see a doctor right away," says Dr. McDuffie. The same goes for a joint that feels stiff, unstable, or numb.

Also be alert to the symptoms of joint infection: warm, swollen, red joints along with fever, chills, or outbreaks of sweating. Unlike RA or osteoarthritis, which progress slowly, an infected joint, left untreated, can go downhill fast. "If you've got an infection, you ought to be in the doctor's office quickly," warns Jeffrey Lisse, M.D., assistant professor of rheumatology at the University of Texas Medical Branch, Galveston. "After a couple of weeks without treatment, the joint could be utterly destroyed."

Where Does It Hurt?

What follows is a guide to joint symptoms in various parts of the body, to help you recognize problems that deserve quick medical attention.

The Back

At some time in our lives, 80 percent of us will experience a backache. In many cases, the problem will go away by itself in a few weeks without medical attention. Most of these backaches are caused by weak or tense muscles. A backache that persists, however, may be caused by arthritis, among other things.

Pain in the lower back or neck may come from osteoarthritis, which causes bone spurs to grow on the spine. Ankylosing spondylitis, a type of arthritis that typically strikes men in their early 20s, causes persistent back pain along with stiffness in the morning. (In a few people, back pain is caused by a "slipped disk," a ruptured vertebral disk that causes pain by pressing on nerves.) Medical tests are necessary to pinpoint the exact cause of a bad back.

According to the *American Medical Association Guide to Back Care,* you should seek medical help for back pain when:

- Your backache lasts more than two weeks.
- The pain shoots down your leg toward your foot or down your arm toward your hand.
- You have numbness or muscle weakness in your leg, foot, arm, or hand.
- Back pain wakes you up at night.
- Back pain is accompanied by problems controlling urination or bowel movements.

The Foot

With more joints than any other part of the body, the foot is a common target of arthritis. In particular, the toe joints are frequent sites of either osteoarthritis or RA. Also, in susceptible people, the big toe can become painfully inflamed with gout. Heel pain, which has a variety of causes, often bothers people with ankylosing spondylitis or Reiter's syndrome, which are other forms of arthritis.

Many people put off getting medical help for foot pain in the mistaken belief that their feet are okay if they can still walk on them. "The truth is that often you can walk with certain types of fractures," says a report from the American Podiatric Medical Association. "Some common examples are breaks of the thinner of the two leg bones, small 'chip' fractures of either foot or ankle bones, and the frequently neglected fracture of a toe."

You should also see a doctor when:

- You notice swelling, heat, and redness in any part of the foot.
- Your foot hurts even when there's no weight on it.
- You sprain your ankle or have any problem that keeps you from walking.
- Your foot is numb in any part.
- You have foot sores that don't heal. (These open wounds could potentially infect the joints.)

But injuries are probably the most common cause of foot pain. Often the problem is a fracture or a soft-tissue injury such as Achilles tendinitis, an inflammation of the heel cord caused by too much running or other activity.

The Knee

The knee is the most injury-prone of all joints. It's also a common site for several kinds of arthritis, including osteoarthritis and infectious arthritis.

See your doctor when:

- Your knee becomes swollen and painful. (Swelling with fever, chills, or a feeling of tiredness may mean an infection.)
- You can't walk on the leg with the affected knee or there is any numbness or loss of feeling in your leg.
- Your knee gives way or is wobbly when you walk or climb stairs.
- Your knee "locks"—it becomes difficult and painful to straighten or bend.

The Elbow

"The most common pains in the elbow are not in the joint. They're in the supporting structures, such as the tendons," says Dr. Lisse. Probably the most common complaint is tennis elbow, a readily treated form of tendinitis. Besides tennis players, people who do certain chores or participate in some hobbies and sports can develop tendinitis of the elbow. The elbow joint itself can be af-fected by several kinds of arthritis, including gout and RA.

See your doctor when:

• You feel pain that does not go away with rest or stopping an overuse activity.

• You have swelling or redness in the elbow or any pain associated with fever and chills.

• You feel a needles-and-pins sensation below a recently injured elbow.

• Your hand becomes cold and painful.

• You feel numbness anywhere in the arm or hand or a lack of pulse at the wrist.

The Shoulder

The shoulder is even more complex than the knee and is ex-tremely susceptible to injuries. "Trauma can result from causes as obvious as a tennis tournament or as subtle as a change in the height of a typing table," according to an article in the journal *Patient Care*. The shoulder joint also can be affected by RA, ankylos-ing spondylitis, and other types of arthritis.

See your doctor when:

• You have swelling or constant pain. "Swelling in the shoulder may be hard to see," says Dr. Lisse. "You may not notice it until it's massive."

• Your shoulder has been injured.

• You have pain that radiates down the arm.

• You feel any numbness or tingling in the shoulder.

• You have trouble lifting your arm out to the side and holding it there.

• You have fever and chills along with pain.

• Your hand becomes cold and painful.

The Hip

The hip is a ball-and-socket joint, which allows the leg to move freely in all directions. Hip pain may be felt in the groin, and often the pain comes not from inside the joint but from a more easily treated inflamed bursa next to the joint. The inner workings of the joint, however, can be hurt by injury or several types of arthritis, including osteoarthritis and ankylosing spondylitis.

See your doctor when:

- Your hip has been recently injured.
- You notice redness, swelling, or persistent pain in the hip.
- You have trouble walking or any problem moving your hips.
- You have fever, chills, or unexplained weight loss along with hip pain.
- You feel weakness, stiffness, numbness, or tingling in the leg.

How to Find a Doctor
Who Understands Arthritis

In most cases, your family doctor is the first person to see if you think you have arthritis. He is the doctor who knows you best and has your medical records.

If you move to a new community or don't have a family doctor, there are several ways to find one. Word of mouth is a good way. Ask a friend or neighbor whose opinion you trust for a recommendation. Another resource is your county medical society, which can provide a list of member physicians. The society also can tell you if a particular doctor has ever had his license restricted or revoked. In addition, many hospitals now have referral hot lines. With a quick call, you can find out about physicians who are on staff or who have privileges at that institution.

If you decide you want to see a specialist in arthritis (a rheumatologist), ask your family doctor for a referral. Or call your local chapter of the Arthritis Foundation for the names of specialists in your area. (See chapter 15, "Who's Who on Your Health Care Team," for more information on arthritis specialists.)

Gather some information before you make an appointment to see a new doctor, advises Dr. Lisse. "The things you want to look for in a doctor are: Did the physician graduate from an accredited medical school? How long has he or she been in practice? Does the doctor impress you as someone who has frequently seen the problems you're complaining about? Does he or she feel comfortable about your getting a second opinion?" Also, find out if the doctor is "board-certified," meaning that he has completed several years of postgraduate training and passed an exam in his specialty.

It's good to stick with a doctor, once you've found one you like, so that a sense of trust and rapport can develop. But if you're dissatisfied with your care, it's okay to discharge your physician and go elsewhere. If possible, first tell your doctor politely why you are unhappy with his care.

"If you start seeing a doctor and over time find out you can't relate to his personality, then you should try to find someone else, because you're going to need the kind of relationship where you can get and give information," says Janet R. Maurer, M.D., assistant professor of medicine at the University of Toronto and author of *How to Talk to Your Doctor: The Questions to Ask.*

Making an Appointment

Getting an appointment to see a busy doctor can be frustrating. If you're worried about your symptoms and can't get a prompt appointment, leave a message to have the doctor call you. Or ask the doctor's office to recommend another physician. Another option: If you live or work within a short distance of the doctor's office, ask to be called if there are any cancellations.

For a sudden and serious joint problem or one that occurs in the middle of the night, go to a hospital emergency room. If you belong to a health maintenance organization, it's wise to check your policy first to find out what its guidelines are for emergency room visits.

Set an Agenda

"Be Prepared" is not just a motto for Boy Scouts. A little planning goes a long way in getting the most out of a doctor's visit—especially considering that many doctors schedule only 15 minutes for the average appointment.

Before you go, spend some time thinking over your symptoms. When did you first start feeling bad? How would you describe your condition? What makes it better or worse? It may help to write down your symptoms and take the list to the office for your personal reference, along with any questions you may have. (See "Ten Questions to Ask Your Doctor about Arthritis" on page 38.)

"Make a list," advises Bruce Hoffman, M.D., associate professor of medicine and chief of rheumatology at the Medical College of Pennsylvania in Philadelphia. "Some doctors laugh when patients come in with lists, but I think it's terrific because, frankly, patients will forget to mention some of their concerns."

"If the patient is prepared and has thought about what's bothering him, it's going to be much easier for me to talk to him about the problem," agrees Dr. Maurer.

The Exam: What to Expect

"How are you?" is the first question you're likely to hear from your doctor. It's natural to want to respond to such a polite query by saying, "Thanks, Doc, I'm fine." But that's not what your doctor wants to hear. ("I usually reply, 'If you were fine, you wouldn't be here,' says Dr. Lisse.) What he's really asking is, "How aren't you? Why did you come to see me? Where does it hurt?"

"You have to struggle with some people to get them to say, 'I'm not fine,' " says Dr. Hoffman, shaking his head.

When you describe your symptoms, be specific. Saying "I have this weird kind of traveling pain that bothers me sometimes," for example, is too vague. More on target: "I get a stabbing pain in my lower back when I bend over or lift a bag of groceries." In other words, explain what the pain feels like, where it hurts, when it occurs, and what seems to make it better.

Don't hesitate to bring up other information about your health, even if you're not sure it's important. A seemingly unrelated pain in your heel, a tingling sensation in your hand, or a case of the blahs all might be important clues to making the diagnosis. "Nobody is going to think you're dumb if you volunteer information," says Dr. Maurer. "At the very worst, the doctor can put your mind to rest by saying that a symptom is nothing to worry about."

Ten Questions to Ask Your Doctor about Arthritis

Doctors don't graduate from medical school with ESP. Preoccupied with other concerns, they can easily overlook health issues that are important to you. If so, there's only one solution: Speak up!

"Information is the basis of everything," says Janet Maurer, M.D., of the University of Toronto. "The more information you have, the better able you will be to handle things."

In general, save questions that require involved answers until the exam is completed, she advises. Most doctors will allow time for five or six questions, she says. A nurse or physical therapist also may be available to field some questions. Try to keep your questions well-organized, easy to follow, and to the point.

Here are ten of the most important questions you can ask about arthritis. Choose the ones that best focus your concerns, or use the list as a springboard to make up your own questions.

1. *What kind of arthritis do I have, and how is it likely to affect me?*

With so many types of arthritis, you need to know which one you have to understand how it will affect you. Ask your doctor to explain your disease and whether you will need to make changes in daily activities.

2. *What will the treatments do, and how long will they take to work?*

Know what to expect. Will there be side effects from drugs? If a particular treatment doesn't work, what are the alternatives?

3. *What can I do to help myself?*

Find out if positive changes in your lifestyle, such as starting a swimming program, are in order. Also, are there self-help devices that can protect your joints around the house or at work?

4. *Do I need to lose weight?*

Being overweight can aggravate some kinds of arthritis. Would losing weight make you feel better? What's a reasonable weight-loss goal?

5. *How will arthritis affect my love life? My family relationships? My social life?*

Arthritis rarely affects only the person who has it. Family members and friends may have to make some adjustments, too, and you'll have to learn how to minimize the impact. Is it okay to remain in the bowling league? To go out dancing? To help your daughter relocate?

6. *What changes in symptoms should I be alert to?*

Can your condition spread to other organs, such as the heart, lungs, or kidneys? If so, be sure you know the warning signs.

7. *How will this affect me financially?*

Any long-term illness can be expensive, and arthritis is no exception. How often will you need to see the doctor? What are the fees for office visits? Lab tests? Hospital care? Are other medications available that offer the same benefits for less money?

8. *Will I be able to work in the same job?*

If you need to change to a less physically demanding job, the sooner you know, the better. That way, you will have plenty of time to plan and learn new skills.

9. *Will I need artificial joints? If so, how successful is joint replacement surgery?*

Usually, surgery to replace joints is an option that comes up later in treatment, and only if other strategies have not worked. Needless to say, surgery is a big decision, one you want to take time to think over. Ask your doctor at what point, if ever, surgery would be recommended.

10. *How do I reach you in an emergency?*

What should you do if an emergency arises in the middle of the night or on a holiday or weekend? Will another physician be available when your doctor is away? Ask for the name of the colleague who covers for your doctor when he is out of town or unavailable.

Solving the Puzzle

Although doctors don't wear trench coats and fedoras, they do think a lot like detectives. Expect lots of questions during the first part of the exam. This process, called the medical history, helps the doctor to identify or rule out various diseases and injuries.

"Think about your conversation with the doctor as a game of Ping-Pong. You give him a symptom, and then you wait for him to ask you a question. Then you respond to his question and wait for him to ask you another question," says a report from the UCLA Medical Center.

Here are some questions to expect if you have symptoms of an arthritic disease.

- Where do you feel your pain?
- Does the pain ever disturb your sleep?
- Is it related to an injury?
- During what part of the 24-hour day is your pain worse?
- Does one side of your body hurt as much as the other?
- Have you had any fever? Chills? Unexplained weight loss?
- Are you taking any medications, including nonprescription drugs?

The doctor also will be interested in your overall health, since many arthritic diseases affect the whole body. "The exam for arthritis is a good, general physical exam," says Richard T. Swanson, M.D., a clinical associate professor of medicine at the Indiana University School of Medicine and head of the rehabilitation unit and services at Welborn Hospital, both in Evansville. "You can't look at the joints out of the context of the whole person."

During the exam, the doctor will check your joints for tenderness and swelling. You may be asked to move parts of your body, with and without the doctor's help. These maneuvers help the doctor find out if your joints can move through their normal range of motion.

Occasionally, some aspect of the exam might be a little surprising or embarrassing. If the doctor suspects you have a joint infection, for example, he may ask if you've had sexual intercourse with a new partner, and he may want to do a pelvic or rectal exam.

The reason: Gonorrhea, a sexually transmitted disease, sometimes infects the joints. He might also check you for tick bites, which can cause a kind of joint pain associated with Lyme disease (discussed in chapter 2, "The Many Faces of Arthritis").

Taking Tests in Stride

Laboratory tests may be necessary to make a diagnosis. You may be asked to give a sample of urine or to have blood or joint fluid drawn for analysis. X rays may be taken of some joints.

X Rays

An X ray is a kind of photograph of the internal structure of a body part. It shows mainly bones, rather than cartilage, muscles, and other soft tissues. Although X rays are widely used, they have some limitations. First, they don't show much in the early stages of RA because the disease causes pain and swelling in the soft tissues long before the bones are damaged. On the other hand, X rays sometimes show early signs of osteoarthritis in people who are feeling fine and don't need treatment.

Many doctors prefer to take X rays of the joints early in treatment, then repeat them at intervals. That way, they can monitor the progress of the disease and watch for any changes in the bones. X rays also are helpful in confirming a diagnosis, especially in someone who has had arthritis for a while.

Blood Tests

Here's a brief rundown of some of the blood tests that your doctor may order to help him in his diagnosis.

Hematocrit and hemoglobin. Both of these tests can detect if you have anemia, or not enough red blood cells. The hematocrit measures the number of red blood cells; hemoglobin is the protein inside these cells that carries oxygen to the tissues from the lungs. People who have RA, lupus, or ankylosing spondylitis are more likely to develop anemia. Also, some medications, such as aspirin, can cause blood to be lost from the digestive tract.

Erythrocyte sedimentation rate. This common test, called the ESR for short, measures whether widespread inflammation is present in the body. A small amount of whole blood is put into a measured cylinder and allowed to settle for an hour. Inflammation is present if the cells drop faster than the standard rate of 20 millimeters (less than 0.1 inch) per hour. In osteoarthritis, the rate is normal. In RA or lupus, the rate is usually high when the disease is active. Your doctor may repeat the test from time to time, because the rate should return to normal as you get better and inflammation subsides.

Uric acid. If your doctor suspects you have gout, he may want to measure the amount of uric acid in your blood. A blood test alone, however, is never enough information to diagnose gout, warns Dr. Hoffman. To be sure, the doctor needs to examine the joint fluid for crystals. (See below.)

Rheumatoid factor. Rheumatoid factor is an abnormal antibody found in many people with RA. But even if a lab test finds you have rheumatoid factor, it does not necessarily mean you have RA, warns Merrill D. Benson, M.D., a professor of medicine and medical genetics in the Rheumatology Division at Indiana University School of Medicine in Indianapolis. Not everybody with RA has this factor. Conversely, some people have the factor but do not have RA.

"The test for rheumatoid factor is one of the most misused of all laboratory tests," states Dr. Benson. "All too often, patients actually free of rheumatoid arthritis may be told they have this disease because of a positive result of the rheumatoid factor test."

This test should be just one part of the diagnosis, along with the medical history, physical exam, and other lab tests, Dr. Benson says.

Joint Fluid Tests

In this common test, a needle is inserted into a joint, usually the knee, and a small amount of fluid is taken out for analysis. "Since the arthritis is going on in the joint, you often learn more from analyzing the joint fluid than you can from analyzing blood tests," says Dr. Benson. This test is usually done by a rheumatologist or orthopedic surgeon. To reduce discomfort, doctors often numb the area first with a local anesthetic such as lidocaine.

By examining the joint fluid, the doctor can look for crystals (a sure sign of gout) or bacteria (a sign of infection). A profusion of white blood cells also indicates that inflammation is present. The same technique sometimes is used to drain excess fluid from a badly swollen joint, relieving stiffness and discomfort.

More Tips for Making the Most of a Doctor Visit

Let's face it: Even Rambo probably gets sweaty palms when he goes to the doctor. It's only natural to worry a little and to feel flustered and distracted. But relax. Here are some tips to help you keep your cool and get as much as possible out of the visit.

Take notes.   Jot down the highlights of what your doctor tells you. It's okay to take notes in the examining room. If you prefer, make your notes right after the visit, perhaps in the waiting room.

Howard MacDonald, who has RA, always keeps a small notebook in his pocket to jot down any changes in his symptoms or questions about his treatment. When he visits his doctor, he refers to the notebook to make sure he hasn't forgotten to discuss anything important. "I might put in a little note to myself, like 'neck aches this week' or 'hands are bothering me.' You've got a lot of things on your mind when you see a doctor, and it's easy to forget those things. This way, I'm sure to remember."

Bring a close friend or family member.   If it would make you feel better, ask someone to accompany you to the doctor's office. Besides helping you to recall important details, a companion provides moral support. "You have an advocate there with you," says Dr. Maurer.

Be assertive.   If you don't understand something, say so. If the doctor uses language that would have confounded Albert Einstein, ask him to repeat it in different words. "The doctor won't be offended if you are assertive," says Dr. Hoffman.

Negotiate.   Find out what your options are. If three different kinds of pills are available to treat inflammation, for example, which one could you take the fewest times a day? Which one is least expensive but just as effective? Work with your doctor to gear your treatment to your needs. After all, no therapy will work if you don't follow it.

Set clear goals for getting better.   Don't leave the office without a clear understanding of what happens next. If you're going to start taking medication, find out when you should begin to feel better and what side effects might show up. Also, find out if more tests will be needed and why. "You should have specific goals because if you don't have specific goals, you have nothing to aim for," says Dr. Maurer.

Getting the Diagnosis

Don't be surprised if you have to visit your doctor several times before he knows exactly what's wrong. Arthritic diseases can be tricky, fooling doctors and patients alike by cleverly masquerading as other illnesses. Sometimes it's necessary to wait until clearer symptoms emerge before a diagnosis can be made.

One young mother consulted four doctors over a two-year period before finally learning she had RA. Shortly after her son was born, she noticed her hands and feet were swollen and painful, especially in the morning. But her first three doctors were puzzled. Her blood tests were normal. And her joint symptoms usually were gone by afternoon, the usual time for her doctors' appointments. "One doctor came in and said, 'There's nothing wrong with you. And besides, you're too pretty to have arthritis.' I was furious!" she recalls. Finally she found a highly regarded rheumatologist, who made the diagnosis after several visits and more tests. Riding the medical merry-go-round was very frustrating in the beginning, says the woman. "But it turned out okay in the end."

"The body is like a good poker player," says Dr. Swanson. "It doesn't show all of its cards at one time."

In the meantime, you and your doctor can work together to devise treatments to make you feel better. And, if you think it would help, get another perspective by going to another doctor for a second opinion.

"If there's a question about the diagnosis, if there's a poor response to therapy, if therapies have been tried and everybody's frustrated, or if it's a life-threatening diagnosis—any of those things are a good reason to get a second opinion," says Dr. Maurer.

Rx for Arthritis:
A Take-Charge Attitude

Okay. You've gone to the doctor. You've padded around in a flimsy hospital robe and your socks. You've been poked and prodded, and you've put up with all kinds of questions. And your suspicions have been confirmed. You have arthritis.

Now what?

The first thing is to get your mind into gear, so your body can get on the mend. "We do know that people with a positive attitude do better," says Dr. McDuffie. Studies at the Stanford Arthritis Center in California show that people with arthritis have less pain and fewer limitations if they feel in charge of their health. Those who think their situation is hopeless fare worse, no matter how much they know about their arthritis.

How can you develop an upbeat attitude in the face of a downer like arthritis? Doctors pass along these tips, gleaned from their happiest patients.

Live your life as normally as possible. Don't fall into a "sick role," advises Dr. Maurer. "A lot of times, people don't realize they can maintain a fairly active life," she says. "And they don't realize they can work actively to overcome the limitations of their disease."

Believe in yourself. "The attitude that 'I'm not going to be beaten by this, and I'm going to do what I'm going to do no matter what,' would be healthy—as long as it doesn't reach the point where you deny you have an illness and don't seek medical attention," says Dr. Hoffman.

Give yourself time to heal. Most types of arthritis progress over years rather than days or weeks. Likewise, you may have to wait several months for some medications to work. Match your expectations to the slow pace of the disease. "You have to be patient," says Dr. Hoffman.

PART

2

The Diet Connection

4

Anatomy of a Healing Diet

For many years, the Arthritis Foundation flatly dismissed any link between diet and arthritis. "The possible relationship between diet and arthritis has been thoroughly and scientifically studied," stated one of the organization's educational pamphlets. "The simple proven fact is: No food has anything to do with causing arthritis and no food is effective in treating or 'curing' it." Most doctors agreed.

But many people with arthritis *disagreed.* "If food has nothing to do with my arthritis," they said, "then why does eating certain foods make my joints feel worse—or better?" Take Phyllis Agard, a homemaker from Massachusetts. She was convinced that drinking coffee made her arthritis worse. But when she shared this observation with her doctor, he was skeptical, to say the least.

"I told him I seemed to be stiff and sore in direct proportion to the amount of coffee I drank," recalls Agard. " 'If you've discovered that caffeine is the cause of arthritis,' he replied sarcastically, 'you've made the discovery of the century.' "

As it turns out, Phyllis Agard (and many others like her) were on the right track. Doctors now say there may be a direct connection between diet and arthritis. (And the Arthritis Foundation recently updated its stance on the food/disease link.) Among the new findings:

- A Detroit doctor has found that people with rheumatoid arthritis (RA) improve dramatically on a low-fat diet.
- Responding to preliminary evidence, researchers at Harvard Medical School and Albany Medical College are testing natural fish oils to find out if they can soothe the inflamed joints of people with RA.
- Doctors at the University of Florida in Gainesville have shown that certain foods, such as dairy products and shrimp, trigger flare-ups of arthritis in a small number of sensitive people.
- Overweight is an important factor in osteoarthritis of the knee, according to Boston University researchers. And slimming down can help relieve the pain of those who already have arthritis, doctors say.

What does this new understanding of food and arthritis mean to you? Should you throw out your aspirin in favor of fish-oil tablets and never eat a fatty food again? Not exactly. You should improve your diet, but do so *gradually* while you continue with your medications and therapy. And make sure your doctor is your partner in planning dietary change.

"I don't think any patient should start out on a diet without first letting the physician know what his plans are," says Michael Weinblatt, M.D., director of the Robert B. Brigham Arthritis Center and assistant professor of medicine at Harvard Medical School, both in Boston.

Okay, you've told your doctor you'd like to consider a healing diet, and he's agreed. What's the next step?

Lean toward Lean

Fat. This calorie-packed nutrient is the great American obsession. Polls show that at any given time, 10 percent of all Americans are on a diet, trying to become trim and thin—or maybe even avoid cancer and circulatory disease, two conditions scientists say may be prevented by low-fat fare. But what even the most fat-conscious Americans probably don't know is that a low-fat diet may help treat RA.

(continued on page 52)

How Fat Is That?

You should try to get about 30 percent or less of your total calories from fat. Compare the foods you now eat with those on the list. If you're eating a lot of foods with more than 30 percent fat, look for good alternatives with less fat. Example: Oil-packed tuna is 37 percent fat, while light-meat tuna packed in water is only 3.4 percent fat.

Fat Content (%)	Foods
0–10	Angel food cake, dried beans and peas, dry cereal, light-meat tuna packed in water, most fruits and vegetables, pretzels, skim milk
10–20	Broiled fish (without butter), roasted chicken (white meat, no skin), sherbet
20–30	Low-fat yogurt, muffins, pancakes, pudding, roasted chicken (dark meat, no skin), roasted turkey
30–40	Broiled chicken (with skin), chocolate cake, fast-food taco, fruit pie, granola, most cookies, oil-packed tuna, 2% milk, waffles

SOURCE: Adapted from *Get Fit!* by Cindy Brown, R.D. (Helena, Mont.: St. Peter's Community Hospital, 1986).

Fat Content (%)	Foods
40–50	Breaded and fried seafood, brownies, donuts, fast-food french fries, fried chicken, pecan pie, regular ice cream, tortilla chips, whole-milk yogurt, whole milk
50–65	Cheesecake, eggs, fast-food fish fillet sandwich, fast-food onion rings, most candy bars, potato chips
65–80	Bacon, cheese, cold cuts, dry-roasted nuts, peanut butter, pork chops, sunflower seeds
Over 80	Butter, cream cheese, light cream, margarine, mayonnaise, oil, salad dressing, sausage, sour cream, shortening

That's the finding of Charles P. Lucas, M.D., clinical professor of medicine at Wayne State University School of Medicine in Detroit and director of the Division of Preventive and Nutritional Medicine at the William Beaumont Hospital in Birmingham, Michigan, who has developed a low-fat diet for his RA patients. People often improve dramatically when they stop eating high-fat dairy products and meat, he says. Instead of these foods, he recommends fish, fruits, vegetables, legumes, grains, skim milk, and low-fat cottage cheese.

"We see the same results over and over again," Dr. Lucas says. "Not everybody, but a significant number of people have a complete reversal or a tremendous improvement in their symptoms. And when they go off the low-fat diet, they usually get worse again."

Dr. Lucas believes the reduction in dietary fats reduces the production of prostaglandins, hormonelike substances that trigger inflammation. Although most doctors don't advocate a low-fat diet for RA, few would argue with the overall health benefits of reducing animal fat, and they would all agree that, within reason, these measures are certainly safe.

Fish Oil: The Good Fat

Not all fat is created equal, however. Meat and dairy products contain *saturated* fat—the bad fat that lards arteries. Fish, however, contain poly*unsaturated* fat, the good fat that helps prevent heart disease. But the fat in fish is better than good—it's downright saintly. Fish oil has a unique group of "fatty acids" (a technical term for a biological component of fat) that scientists have dubbed omega-3's. Research shows that omega-3's may help stop cholesterol buildup, slow some types of cancer, lower blood pressure, prevent blood clots—and possibly treat RA and lupus.

Omega-3 fatty acids are thought to work on these last two diseases by reducing the body's production of prostaglandins and leukotrienes, hormonelike substances that turn on inflammation in the joints and other tissues. Cold-water ocean fish, such as salmon, tuna, and mackerel, are especially rich sources of omega-3's. That may be why Eskimos, who eat lots of fish, rarely get RA and the other illnesses that fish oils seem to protect against.

"I recommend to all my patients that they eat more fish because I think there is overwhelming evidence that eating more fish is good for people," says Joel M. Kremer, M.D., associate professor of medicine at Albany Medical College.

Dr. Kremer and his colleagues found that taking fish-oil capsules helped to soothe painful joints in people with RA. Twenty patients took 15 fish-oil pills (an amount of oil roughly equal to that in 8 ounces of mackerel) daily for 14 weeks, while a second group took look-alike capsules that didn't contain oil. At the end of 14 weeks, the group taking fish oil had fewer painful joints and less fatigue. Even after they switched to the fake pills after 14 weeks, they continued to show some improvement.

"For the first time, we have demonstrated that a dietary manipulation can favorably affect RA," says Dr. Kremer. "It's remarkable to be able to say that."

In another study at Harvard Medical School, 12 RA patients took 20 fish-oil pills daily for ten weeks, while a second group took olive oil. At the end of six weeks, the patients taking fish oil had fewer painful joints and other signs of inflammation than the patients who took olive oil.

Dr. Weinblatt, a researcher in the Harvard study, says the results are encouraging but cautions that fish oil may have only modest benefits compared to established treatments. "It may not be as good as aspirin as an anti-inflammatory agent," he says. "Or maybe, at best, it will be as good." Another doctor adds that fish oil, when used along with conventional therapy for arthritis, may enhance the benefits of the treatment.

The most natural way to get more omega-3 fatty acids is to eat more fish. (See "Omega-3 Content of Fish" on page 54.) A daily serving of 6 ounces of sardines in oil, for example, would give you more omega-3 fatty acids than were used in Dr. Kremer's study. "What you'd pay for ten capsules is what you'd pay for a can of sardines," he says. "You'd get more fish oil from the sardines, and they're better for you."

Donald A. Rudin, M.D., author of *The Omega-3 Phenomenon,* recommends eating several pounds of cold-water ocean fish each

Omega-3 Content of Fish	
Fish (6 oz.)	Omega-3 Fatty Acids (g)
Mackerel, Atlantic	4.4
Mackerel, king	3.7
Herring, Pacific	3.1
Herring, Atlantic	2.9
Tuna, bluefin	2.7
Sablefish	2.6
Salmon, chinook	2.6
Sturgeon, Atlantic	2.6
Tuna, albacore	2.6
Whitefish, lake	2.6
Anchovies, European	2.4
Salmon, Atlantic	2.4
Salmon, sockeye	2.2
Bluefish	2.0
Mullet	1.9
Salmon, coho	1.7
Salmon, pink	1.7

week. If you're looking for creative ways to add fish to your diet, take a few tips from the Rudin family. "We've increased our fish intake to practically three dinners a week," says Dr. Rudin's wife, Joan. "We have smoked salmon for breakfast, which is delightful. We eat tuna fish for lunch or often have it for dinner." And for snacks, the Rudins munch on mackerel from tins.

If you do decide to take the capsules, which are available without prescription from supermarkets, pharmacies, and health food stores, consider this: In Dr. Kremer's study, several patients got stomachaches from the pills. Some burped more than usual and got a fishy taste in the mouth. Also, fish oil thins blood. (That's why it's good for those with heart disease.) Consult your doctor first about avoiding or reducing unwanted effects.

Dr. Rudin and other doctors advise against taking cod-liver oil for arthritis. Although this home remedy is a rich source of omega-3's, it also is high in vitamins A and D, which can become toxic if taken in high doses for a long period of time. If you feel you must take cod-liver oil, never take more than 1 teaspoon a day, advises Dr. Rudin.

Although less well known as sources of omega-3's, certain vegetable oils also contain rich amounts. Researchers aren't sure, however, whether or not plant sources have the same health benefits as fish.

The Vitamin Connection: Hype or Help?

It's an arthritis victim's dream: a vitamin pill that will banish aches and pains. Yet for every study published in a major journal showing that a particular nutrient improves some form of arthritis, another report comes along and contradicts the findings. Here's the latest on six nutrients that may—or may not—help. (You should undertake a supplement program only with the approval and supervision of your doctor.)

Vitamin C. A few studies show that vitamin C can slow the development of osteoarthritis in animals. The studies were done in guinea pigs, which, like humans, must get their vitamin C from their diet. The guinea pigs underwent a type of surgery that caused them to develop osteoarthritis of the knee. Guinea pigs fed low amounts of vitamin C (enough to protect against scurvy) developed severe osteoarthritis, but those fed higher-than-normal amounts had very little arthritis.

"Our interpretation is that vitamin C, under this disease state, does have a protective role," says Edith R. Schwartz, Ph.D., professor of orthopedics and physiology at Tufts University School of Medicine in Boston, who conducted the studies. "It does not cure osteoarthritis, but it can serve a protective role."

"If you have arthritis, you certainly should not let yourself get low on vitamin C," Dr. Schwartz says. Good sources are citrus fruits, strawberries, green peppers, mustard greens, and tomatoes. The Recommended Dietary Allowance of vitamin C is about 60 milligrams. If you're considering supplements, it's wise to check with your doctor before taking excess vitamin C to make sure it won't interfere with your care.

Vitamin E. Vitamin E and vitamin C work together as partners in the fight against chemicals that break down joint cartilage, Dr. Schwartz has found. She believes vitamin E may also be helpful in slowing osteoarthritis. The Recommended Dietary Allowance of vitamin E is 10 milligrams. (There are several forms of vitamin E, and dosage is sometimes expressed in international units. One synthetic form, for example, has 1.1 international units per milligram, while some naturally occurring forms have about 1.5 international units per milligram.) The best sources are corn oil, sunflower seeds, wheat germ, nuts, whole grains, and legumes.

Copper. "Copper treatment for rheumatoid arthritis began with use of copper bracelets among the ancient Greeks," writes Richard S. Panush, M.D., in *Rehabilitation and Management of Rheumatic Conditions.* "Copper was considered to have a mysterious power to relieve aches and pains." People with RA have higher-than-normal levels of copper in their blood, and copper levels tend to go *up* when people feel worse and fall when they get better. Most doctors, however, believe the disturbed copper levels have *nothing* to do with causing or treating the disease. Most people need about 2 milligrams of copper daily. The best sources are oysters and soybeans. (Copper bracelets are discussed in chapter 16, "Alternative Remedies: Proceed with Caution.")

Zinc. People with RA—an autoimmune disease—often have low levels of zinc, which is necessary for a healthy immune system. In one study, people with RA improved after taking zinc supplements. The patients, who took 220 milligrams of zinc three times a day for 12 weeks, had less pain, joint swelling, and morning stiffness. Unfortunately, the role of zinc remains cloudy, because other researchers have not duplicated these findings. And the people in this study took several hundred milligrams more of this nutrient than the average diet provides or requires.

You need only about 15 milligrams of zinc daily. Seven ounces of oysters, by far the richest source, has 150 milligrams. Other good sources are ground beef, veal, pork, shrimp, fish, soybeans, granola, cheddar cheese, and tofu.

Selenium. Getting too little selenium, a trace mineral, causes a rare type of premature and disabling arthritis called

Kashin-Beck disease. The amount of selenium in foods varies with the selenium content of soil. That's probably the reason that Kashin-Beck disease is most common in areas of China where the soil is poor in selenium. Fortunately, this type of arthritis occurs rarely, if ever, in the United States, where selenium-containing foods are abundant.

You need between 50 and 200 micrograms of selenium daily. Good sources are fish and meat, as well as grains, legumes, and nuts.

Calcium. While everyone needs to get enough calcium in their diet, people with RA should be doubly careful because they are more likely to lose calcium from their bones, especially if they take corticosteroids. When the bones lose calcium, they become porous and fragile, a condition known as osteoporosis.

The Recommended Dietary Allowance for calcium is between 1,000 and 1,500 milligrams daily; the higher amount is for women who are past menopause. A cup of milk contains about 300 milligrams of calcium. Other good sources are cheese, dark leafy greens, canned sardines, tofu, cottage cheese, soybeans, broccoli, and legumes. Postmenopausal women who have trouble getting their full quota of calcium from dietary sources may be candidates for estrogen replacement, which can help their bodies hang on to the calcium they do get.

If you don't always eat as well as you'd like, you can get the recommended allowance of many missing nutrients from a daily multivitamin pill. "A lot of people feel like they want to do something extra for themselves. If you're going to do anything for yourself, a daily vitamin is the safest and best thing to do," says Linda Zorn Newcomb, a registered dietitian who is coordinator of the National Wellness Association (membership division), which has its headquarters in Stevens Point, Wisconsin.

Fewer Pounds, Less Pain

If you consult a doctor for your arthritis, the first advice you're apt to hear is, "Lose weight." Shedding extra pounds reduces stress on your aching joints, especially if you have arthritis in weight-bearing joints such as your knees, back, or hips. Weight control also is helpful if you have gout, because it may lower levels of uric acid in the blood.

"If a person is more than 30 pounds overweight, it is necessary to reduce," says Nancy Holden, who works with arthritis patients at the Division of Preventive and Nutritional Medicine of the William Beaumont Hospital in Birmingham, Michigan. "Once you take a lot of the weight off the joints, people feel tremendously better. We've had patients come in who were going to have knee surgery or hip surgery. Well, as soon as the weight was gone, they no longer needed surgery," she says. (In fact, many surgeons will not replace joints until weight is lost because excess weight causes excess wear on the new artificial joint.)

Besides overburdening sensitive joints, being overweight is an important cause of arthritis of the knee. That conclusion was drawn from information from the ongoing Framingham Heart Study in Massachusetts. Boston University researchers studied two groups of older Framingham citizens, with and without arthritis of the knee. When the researchers looked at data from when the people were in their mid-30s, they found that those with arthritis had been significantly heavier than those without the problem. Overweight was a more important cause of this type of arthritis in women than in men, says David T. Felson, M.D., one of the researchers and an assistant professor of medicine at Boston University School of Medicine.

How do extra pounds lead to arthritis of the knee? "One of the most likely theories is the one that makes the most sense—that increased weight leads to increased force on the joints," says Dr. Felson. In other words, the joint cartilage eventually breaks down when burdened with a too-heavy load. But that's just one of several theories. Other researchers speculate that a weight problem may cause subtle changes in the body's chemistry, perhaps unleashing factors in the blood that harm the joints. That theory is somewhat supported by the fact that a weight problem also can lead to osteo-arthritis of the hands, which obviously aren't weight-bearing joints.

Losing weight is not easy for anyone, and that's especially true if you have arthritis. If your joints are painful and stiff, it's tempting to forgo exercise. That sets up a vicious cycle. If you don't stay active and exercise your joints, you may feel stiffer. That in turn perpetuates more inactivity— and more weight gain, since you'll burn fewer calories if you spend most of your time in cars, on a chair or the couch, or in bed.

Take a Good Look at Yourself

So what have you got to lose? Honest self-appraisal is the best way to answer that question. Look at your body candidly in a full-length mirror or study yourself in some recent photographs. One picture is worth a thousand height/weight charts.

Here's a quick calculation to determine your ideal weight from Sarah L. Morgan, M.D., a registered dietitian and an instructor in clinical nutrition and preventive medicine at the University of Alabama in Birmingham. For a woman, take 100 pounds for your first 5 feet of height, then add 5 pounds for each additional inch of height. If you are 5-feet-8-inches tall, for example, you should weigh roughly 140 pounds, or 100 plus 40 (5 pounds times 8 inches). For a man, take 106 pounds for your first 5 feet of height, then add 6 pounds for each additional inch.

If you do decide to go on a diet, check with your physician to make sure your health is up to it. The next step is to adopt a winning—or losing—attitude.

"Beginning a diet is not a prison sentence," says Judy Walthaw, a registered dietitian who works with arthritis patients at the University of Alabama Hospitals in Birmingham. "Don't deny yourself all foods or eat less often. Instead, try focusing on foods that give the most essential nutrients for the least calories."

To lose weight, you needn't turn into a "calorie cost accountant," tallying up the calories in every bite. "For you to maintain your weight for a lifetime, your diet has to be something that will fit into your lifestyle and be easy to do," says registered dietitian Bettye Nowlin, a spokeswoman for the American Dietetic Association. "Counting calories is just not realistic."

Instead, make some simple changes in your eating habits. Cut down on the size of portions. Eat more slowly to give foods a chance to satisfy your hunger. Listen to your stomach; try to concentrate on eating when you're hungry and stopping when you're

(continued on page 62)

Exorcise Your Diet Demons

Everyone has his own personal diet demons—emotional gremlins that trick you into eating when you don't really want to. Others have mindless hand-to-mouth nibbling habits they just can't break. Bettye Nowlin, spokeswoman for the American Dietetic Association, offers these helpful hints for recognizing what makes you eat too much—and for controlling your appetite.

The Enemy	Your Defense
You head straight for the refrigerator when you come home from work.	Curb your appetite by bringing an apple or a banana to eat on the way home.
You nosh constantly on cookies and candy to relieve tension at work.	Keep crisp, raw, low-calorie veggies handy to crunch on.
When you're at a party, you can't stop nibbling at the buffet.	Socialize. Set a goal to talk to two new people. You can't talk with your mouth full!
You feel compelled to eat every morsel on your plate; your mother said people were starving.	People are starving somewhere, but you're not. Write a check for a famine-relief charity and toss or save your leftovers.
You snack mindlessly while watching television.	Keep your hands busy with something other than food. Knit, write a letter, manicure your nails, give your spouse a back rub.

The Enemy	Your Defense
You eat after fighting with someone you love.	Get out of the house. Soothe your anger with something other than food. Window-shop, take a drive, or go to a movie.
You eat when you feel lonely or blue.	Call a friend. Find a buddy to exercise with. Join an outing club or volunteer group that widens your circle of friends.
You can't resist the temptation of your favorite sinful dessert.	Splurge once in a while. Enjoy a small amount to satisfy your craving.
You're too pooped to cook so you eat greasy fast foods.	Look for a lighter fast-food fare. Try Mexican, Chinese, or pizza without sausage.

full. (If you often overeat because you're angry or stressed or for other emotional reasons, see "Exorcise Your Diet Demons" on page 60.)

And join the fat patrol. Hunt down and eliminate fatty foods in your diet by keeping a food diary for a week. At the end of the week, sit down and circle all the fatty and high-calorie foods in your notebook—butter, margarine, cream, most cheeses and dairy products (except those clearly labeled "low-fat" or "nonfat"), fatty cuts of meat, baked goods, candy, and sauces. Read labels. Next to your circled foods, jot down lighter versions of the same food. Substitute puffed wheat cereal for granola, for example. Have a Popsicle instead of an ice cream bar. Try vegetable soup instead of cream soup with milk. Often, you can simply cook the same food differently. Steaming, baking, and broiling without fat are better than frying.

Here are more hints for successful weight control.

- If an irresistible urge to eat strikes, set a 3-minute timer and wait for it to go off before you cave in, suggests Dr. Morgan. By then you may have reconsidered, she says. "If you want to go and eat after that, that's fine."
- Divide and conquer. If you want to lose 20 pounds, break that into four goals of 5 pounds each. Reward yourself each time you meet a mini-goal with a massage, a new sweater, or some other nonfood splurge.
- Don't fast or crash diet. Aim for a gradual weight loss of about 2 pounds a week. Trying to lose weight too fast may slow your metabolism, making it even harder to lose. Also, if you have gout, crash dieting can raise uric acid levels and trigger an attack.
- Don't weigh yourself every day. If you hit a temporary plateau, you may get discouraged and give up. Weighing yourself once a week is fine.
- Get more exercise. You will lose weight faster and feel better if you exercise as part of your weight-loss plan. Most important, you'll lose fat, not muscle. (Guidelines for planning an exercise program are outlined in part 3, "Move Away from Pain.")

CHAPTER

5

Alternative Arthritis Diets

"Let Chinese Bug Juice Banish Your Aches and Pains," declares a headline, aimed at arthritis sufferers, in a supermarket tabloid. "Eat cherries!" urges a book of folk remedies. "A Miracle in Arizona: Finally there is real hope for those who suffer from arthritis," screams an advertisement for a vitamin supplement.

From every possible direction, people with arthritis are bombarded with nutritional information—and misinformation. It's hard for a sane person to know what to eat. One diet promises relief if you don't eat eggplant, peppers, potatoes, and tomatoes. Another advises you to eat raw liver and avoid flour in any form. Yet another recommends drinking a solution of apple cider vinegar and honey twice a day.

People with arthritis spend up to a billion dollars a year in search of relief—much of it for worthless diet information. No wonder the Arthritis Foundation has cautioned the public about dietary quick fixes for so many years.

Can any of these diets *really* relieve arthritis? Not long ago, if you asked your doctor that question, you'd get a firm and thunderous, "No!" Lacking convincing scientific evidence, doctors were understandably skeptical of a diet/arthritis connection. If you felt better from diet changes, the benefit was said to be a "placebo" effect—you felt better simply because you expected to. Or the improvement was attributed to coincidence, since people with arthritis normally feel better at some times and worse at others.

But in light of recent findings, many doctors have begun to pay more attention to arthritis-relief diets. Should *you* try some of the diets? That depends. If you've never noticed a connection between your arthritis and food—and many people don't—then eat your normal diet in peace. On the other hand, if you have a hunch that a certain food makes your arthritis better or worse, go ahead and investigate, says Robert M. Stroud, M.D., clinical professor of medicine at the University of Florida College of Medicine in Gainesville.

If you do plan an expedition through the sometimes wild jungle of arthritis diets, use this chapter to help you distinguish sensible advice from nonsense.

Food Sensitivity
May Be the Culprit

Connie Gregory is a 31-year-old mother who has had rheumatoid arthritis (RA) since she was 17. She's learned to live without beef, pork, caffeine, and sweets. Through careful observation, she has discovered that these foods invariably make her arthritis worse.

"I'd eat those foods, and within a few hours to a day, my joints would swell up," says Gregory, who lives in Tremont, Illinois. "Sometimes I literally could not walk. It was that dramatic."

Gregory's story is what researchers call "anecdotal" evidence of a link between food sensitivity and arthritis. Although people with arthritis have been saying for years that certain foods can trigger flare-ups, it wasn't until recently that researchers confirmed the relationship in scientific tests.

One of the scientists credited for bringing this subtle connection to light is Richard S. Panush, M.D., chief of the Division of Clinical Immunology, Rheumatology, and Allergy at the University of Florida College of Medicine. "There is compelling evidence suggesting that some patients who have rheumatic diseases may indeed be diet- or food-sensitive," states Dr. Panush in *Arthritis and Rheumatism.*

But the real unsung heroine of this story is one of Dr. Panush's patients. To protect her privacy, researchers call her P. S., but this 52-year-old woman has earned a place in medical history books. P. S., who has RA, knew her arthritis got worse after ingesting milk, red meat, dry beans, and some other foods. To prove her point, she volunteered to become a human guinea pig.

P. S. was one of the first patients to pass the "double-blind" test for food-sensitive arthritis—medical science's ultimate proof. In a double-blind study, neither the subject nor the investigators know whether a placebo or the real test substance is being given. P. S., who agreed to stay in the hospital for the study, first fasted for three days to clear her system of any residue of food. She then began eating a formula diet free of allergenic foods. The researchers then "challenged" P. S. by giving her capsules containing a variety of dried foods.

The results were dramatic: When P. S. took capsules containing lettuce or carrots, her symptoms were unchanged. But when she took capsules containing dried milk, she became much worse—exactly as she had when she was careless about her diet.

"This is a landmark study, which shows [food-allergic arthritis] does exist," says Dr. Stroud, one of the investigators. "The next logical step is to find out who is allergic and how to diagnose them simply."

P. S. may be the best example of a case of food-allergic arthritis, but she's not alone in the medical literature. In one case report, a dermatologist traced his arthritis to sodium nitrate, found in cured ham, smoked salmon, and his favorite Cervelat sausage. Other foods linked to arthritis in some patients include corn, beef, wheat, and dairy products, says Dr. Stroud. (As with medications, however, what works for one patient may not necessarily work for others.)

How Foods Can Trigger Arthritis

Scientists aren't sure yet how food can trigger an arthritis flare-up. The best hypothesis is that food molecules slip through the lining of the intestine and enter the bloodstream. When the food molecules reach the joints, they become stuck to the surface of mast cells, components of the body's immune system. When the mast cells latch onto the food molecules, they detonate like microscopic bombs, showering the joint (or other tissues) with inflammation-causing chemicals.

Symptoms of food-sensitive arthritis differ from person to person. Dr. Stroud recalls one woman whose joints swelled dramatically within 10 minutes of eating a grapefruit. Others have a delayed reaction, with symptoms peaking a day or two after eating a certain food—which makes it much harder to pinpoint the suspect food.

How many people with arthritis can blame their achy joints on something they eat? Estimates vary widely. According to Dr. Panush, less than 5 percent of people with RA have symptoms connected to foods. But Dr. Stroud believes the problem is much more common, especially among people with RA. He estimates up to 40 percent of RA patients have food-aggravated arthritis.

And so far, doctors have confirmed food-sensitive flare-ups in only a few people with RA and a few with lupus. Scientists don't know yet if people with other types of arthritis also may have food-related episodes.

How to Find Out If Your Joints Are Allergic

If you have a hunch that a particular food may be triggering your symptoms, here are some guidelines to help you uncover the connection.

• Keep a "bad-day" diary, suggests Dr. Stroud. Write down everything you ate in the 24 hours preceding a flare-up. By comparing what you ate before several episodes, you may be able to identify the likely culprit.

• If you suspect a food does bother you, stop eating it for at least five days to give it time to exit your system. Then try the food again and see if your symptoms get worse. If you repeat this test twice and your symptoms get worse each time, you can be reasonably sure there's a connection.

- Think twice before you banish any food from your diet. If it's something you don't eat often, such as shrimp or strawberries, you probably won't miss it. But don't give up a major food group, such as dairy products or grains, unless you're sure you can get the nutrients they provide from other foods.
- However, if you decide to cut out something more than an occasional food, work with your doctor and, ideally, a dietitian. Diets that successfully manage a food allergy can be tricky even for experienced professionals because of time lags between eating a food and having a flare-up.

Another Potential Pain Reliever: Tryptophan

Eliminating an allergenic food may help reduce pain and inflammation in your joints. But you may want to bring your arthritis complaints to a higher authority: your brain, the master organ for controlling pain sensitivity.

For years, scientists thought our brains existed in a state of splendid isolation, supremely indifferent to changes in diet. Researchers now say that nutrients found in ordinary foods *can* subtly change the brain's chemistry—helping you to feel more cheerful, sleep better, and ward off pain.

For people with chronic pain, one of the most important of these nutritional tranquilizers is tryptophan (sometimes labeled L-tryptophan). Tryptophan is an amino acid, a natural component of the protein in milk, meat, eggs, and other foods. In your brain, tryptophan is converted into a neurotransmitter, or nerve messenger, called serotonin.

Serotonin works like a chemical lullaby. When levels are high—when plenty of tryptophan is around—serotonin can quell chronic pain and chase away insomnia and the blues. "Tryptophan is the key that turns the serotonin lock," writes Robert L. Pollack, Ph.D., a professor of biochemistry and chairman of the Department of Chemistry and Nutrition at Temple University School of Dentistry in Philadelphia, who is author of *The Pain-Free Trypto-*

phan Diet. "Without adequate amounts of tryptophan in the diet, you cannot make and maintain the vital level of serotonin that is so essential to your overall good health and to controlling and regulating pain."

At the school of dentistry, Dr. Pollack and Samuel Seltzer, D.D.S., showed the pain-fighting power of tryptophan. In one of several studies, 15 people with head or neck pain received daily capsules of tryptophan to boost their levels of serotonin. Another 15 patients received a placebo pill. After eight days, the tryptophan group felt less pain than the control group. It also felt more rested, relaxed, and in better spirits, Dr. Pollack says.

Unfortunately, tryptophan has not been well studied as a pain-fighter for arthritis. However, Richard M. Linchitz, M.D., medical director of the Pain Alleviation Center in Roslyn, New York, and author of *Life without Pain,* sometimes recommends tryptophan supplements to his patients with arthritis. The nutrient works as well for various types of arthritis as it does for other chronic pain, he says. "It's usually worth a try. When it's added to a whole program of therapy, it seems to be a benefit."

If you eat an average American diet, you already consume about 2 grams of tryptophan daily. It's found in milk, poultry, and other high-protein foods. However, tryptophan is a fussy nutrient. It won't work well unless your diet is carefully balanced. For one thing, tryptophan doesn't like too much fat. In the blood, tryptophan piggybacks on circulating blood proteins, and too much fat can knock tryptophan off its ride, preventing it from reaching the brain. Aim for no more than 30 percent of your total calories from fat. Try to get most of your calories from complex carbohydrates, such as fruits, vegetables, grains, and cereals, says Dr. Pollack.

One more thing. Although tryptophan comes from protein, it competes with its fellow amino acids. So if you eat too much protein, the resulting swarm of other amino acids can bump tryptophan from the transport system that normally carries it into the brain. Try to get between 10 and 15 percent of your total calories from protein. That's about 6 to 8 ounces of meat a day, depending on your size. (Women usually need less than men.)

Within a few months, some people will feel better simply by making these changes in their diet, Dr. Pollack says.

A Word of Caution about Tryptophan Capsules

To get a greater boost from this antipain nutrient, some people take tryptophan supplements. (Because of tryptophan's powerful effect on the brain, however, supplements act more like a drug than a food. For that reason, it's essential to consult your physician before taking tryptophan capsules.) Tryptophan is available without a prescription in health food stores and pharmacies. Dr. Pollack says, "Look for capsules that also contain niacin and vitamin B_6, which create the optimal working environment for tryptophan in the body."

According to Dr. Linchitz, tryptophan works best if you spread the dose out over the day. The average tablet contains 500 milligrams. Doctors who prescribe this treatment suggest their patients try four tablets daily for a total of 2 grams. One way would be to take a tablet with breakfast, one with lunch, one with dinner, and one before bedtime with a banana or other carbohydrate snack. "Take the smallest amount that will do the job," advises Dr. Pollack. After two or three weeks, begin to taper off the supplements. In Dr. Pollack's studies, people needed smaller maintenance doses as time passed.

To play it safe, don't take more than 2 grams of tryptophan a day. Michael Trulson, Ph.D., former associate professor of anatomy at Texas A&M University, has found that high doses of tryptophan cause liver damage in rats. Although this finding has not been confirmed by other studies, and Dr. Pollack and Dr. Linchitz have not seen this problem in people, all agree it's wise to be cautious. If you take the supplements, ask your doctor about liver function tests, Dr. Linchitz suggests.

Also, never give tryptophan supplements to infants or children, and don't take them yourself if you are pregnant or have asthma. Further, Dr. Trulson says tryptophan should not be used by people diagnosed as having Addison's disease or other problems of the adrenal cortex.

The most common side effect of taking tryptophan is sleepiness, since serotonin is involved in sleep pathways. Although other side effects are uncommon, Dr. Linchitz suggests you stop taking the supplements and consult further with your physician if you begin to experience increased fatigue, runny or stuffed nose, intestinal cramps or constipation, or extreme nervousness.

Dr. Dong's Arthritis Diet from China

When modern American medicine failed to help his crippling arthritis, Collin H. Dong, M.D., returned to his ancient roots and found relief in a simple Chinese diet.

At age 35, Dr. Dong was afflicted with a baffling form of arthritis that seemed hopeless. Although he consulted many specialists and took powerful medications, his arthritis became progressively worse. Growing desperate, Dr. Dong suddenly recalled an ancient Chinese proverb that he believes eventually saved him: "Sickness enters through the mouth, and catastrophe comes out of the mouth."

"Incredible as it may sound, this axiom was the straw that eventually rescued me from a wheelchair," he writes in *The Arthritic's Cookbook.* "Perhaps I had been putting some 'sickness' through my mouth for a long time without realizing it."

In short, Dr. Dong blamed the typical American diet—full of red meat, fat, additives, and preservatives—for his arthritis. Dr. Dong, who had stopped eating the Chinese diet of his youth during his medical training, believed his illness was an allergic reaction to the American diet. To test his hypothesis, he switched back to the traditional Chinese diet of mostly fish, vegetables, and rice.

"To my utter amazement, in a few short weeks there was a metamorphosis," he writes. "I was agile again, for I went from 195 to 150 pounds. I was able to play golf again, for the stiffness and pain in my joints disappeared. I was able to smile again, for the psychological torture of years was alleviated. I had almost a complete remission from my crippling disease."

Despite the skepticism of his medical colleagues, Dr. Dong went on to tell the world about his diet. In his book, he claims to have treated thousands of cases of arthritis. "The high percentage of remissions from pain and misery with my method is remarkable," he writes.

Was the well-meaning doctor on to something? A few years ago, the Dong diet was put to the test by Dr. Panush and his colleagues at the University of Florida. Fifteen patients with RA followed the Dong diet for ten weeks, while another group ate a control diet. Five patients improved on the Dong diet. However, six patients on a control diet also got better, which means it's hard to determine if the Dong diet had any special effect.

Nonetheless, two patients on the Dong diet improved substantially and chose to stick with the diet when the experiment ended. When these patients eat certain foods forbidden by the Dong diet, their arthritis gets worse, reports Dr. Panush.

Apparently the Dong diet does benefit some people with arthritis. And even if it doesn't help your joints, the Dong diet is reasonably healthful, since it is low in cholesterol and saturated fats. Since meat and dairy products are excluded, however, the diet can be low in calcium and some other nutrients. In Dr. Panush's study, some participants took a daily multivitamin with iron to supply essential nutrients.

Do's and Don'ts on the Dong Diet

If you want to try the Dong diet, follow these basic guidelines.

Foods allowed: All seafood except sardines; all vegetables except tomatoes; vegetable oil; soybean margarine; egg whites; oatmeal; cream of wheat; grits; any kind of flour; sugar, honey, maple syrup, or corn syrup; all kinds of rice; bread without preservatives; tea and coffee; and plain soda water.

Foods not allowed: Meat; meat broth; fruit; dairy products; egg yolks; vinegar; pepper; chocolate; dry roasted nuts; alcoholic beverages; soft drinks; and all additives, preservatives, and chemicals (with the exception of lecithin in margarine).

Foods allowed occasionally: Chicken breast; chicken broth; a small amount of wine in cooking; a pinch of spicy seasoning; and noodles and pasta.

The Feel-Good Vegetarian Diet

It won't cure your arthritis, but a vegetarian diet may make you feel better, reports one Swedish researcher.

Lars Sköldstam, of the Department of Internal Medicine at Sundsvalls Hospital in Sundsvall, Sweden, found that 60 percent of RA patients who followed a vegan diet (a vegetarian diet that allows no animal products of any kind) said they felt less pain and were better able to function.

The 20 patients, who first fasted for seven to ten days, eliminated meat, dairy products, strong spices, alcohol, tea, and coffee. They also used little or no refined sugar, corn flour, or salt. They continued taking their arthritis medications as usual.

After four months as vegans, 12 reported they felt better, 5 were unchanged, and 3 were worse. A pleasant side effect: Nearly all the patients lost extra weight. The diet also was virtually free of cholesterol and had plenty of healthful polyunsaturated fats.

Sköldstam isn't sure how the diet works, and he found no evidence that the diet lessened the underlying disease. Objective measurements, such as joint tenderness, grip strength (a measure of hand squeeze), and blood tests, all were unchanged. He concluded that "many patients with mild or moderate rheumatoid arthritis benefit from eating the vegan diet in that they will feel subjectively better. However, the diet does not seem to significantly suppress the rheumatoid disease to any significant extent."

Sköldstam speculates that the change in dietary fats might play a role in reducing inflammation, and he isn't the first to suggest a vegetarian diet for people with arthritis. At least five other authors have written popular books on the subject. If you're considering a vegetarian diet, here are some guidelines to keep in mind.

• If you give up meat, your diet may lack iron, zinc, and some of the B vitamins provided by meat. You can get more of these nutrients by eating legumes, tofu, prunes, peas, raisins, nuts, granola, and whole wheat products.

• If you omit eggs and dairy products as well as meat, you can run short of vitamin B_{12}, a nutrient found only in animal foods. Consider a vitamin B_{12} supplement or drink soymilk or a similar product fortified with vitamin B_{12}.

• If you choose to omit all animal products, you'll also need more protein-rich plant foods, such as legumes and nuts. Some examples are peanuts, whole wheat bread, rice, beans (especially soybeans), corn, and pasta (or combinations of these foods).

• Without dairy products, you also may get too little calcium, increasing your risk of osteoporosis. Consider a calcium supplement, and try to get more of this mineral by eating more dark leafy greens such as kale, turnip greens, mustard greens, and collard greens, as well as tofu, soybeans, and other legumes.

Should You "Just Say No" to Nightshades?

What would spaghetti be without tomato sauce? Or a burger without french fries? People who follow the "no-nightshades" diet soon find out. This diet forbids familiar foods like potatoes, eggplant, tomatoes, and peppers—all members of the botanical family called nightshades. (Those who follow the diet also are advised to stop smoking because tobacco is a nightshade plant.)

This diet was developed by Norman F. Childers, Ph.D., a now-retired Rutgers University horticulture professor who believed that the nightshade family of plants was directly responsible for the aches and pains of most cases of arthritis.

His rationale: Nightshades contain a substance called solanine, which, according to Dr. Childers, is a natural poison that causes arthritis in sensitive people by slowly poisoning them.

Most nutritional experts disagree with Dr. Childers. Although solanine is a toxin and is found in nightshade foods, it's present in such tiny amounts that you couldn't possibly eat enough to do yourself any harm, says Patricia Giblin Wolman, Ed.D., a registered dietitian and associate professor of human nutrition and food systems management at Winthrop College in Rock Hill, South Carolina. Another issue that hasn't been addressed is whether people in areas where these foods are eaten regularly—in Ireland or Italy, for example—have more arthritis.

Nevertheless, some people with arthritis say the diet helps them. Dr. Childers surveyed more than 1,000 volunteers who followed his diet and found that 70 percent experienced some relief after avoiding the nightshades. The diet is nutritionally sound, although it eliminates some good sources of vitamins A and C. (Apricots, carrots, cantaloupe, spinach, sweet potatoes, and winter squash are alternate sources of vitamin A. Cauliflower, citrus fruits, and strawberries are alternate sources of vitamin C.)

To follow the diet to the letter, you have to give up such all-American favorites as beef stew (potatoes), clam chowder (potatoes), baked beans (tomatoes), barbecued chicken (tomatoes), and ketchup. No chili either—spices such as chili powder, paprika, and cayenne are all derived from peppers. Also, you need to check the labels of processed foods carefully to find hidden sources of potatoes and tomatoes. If you're willing to put up with these severe restrictions in hope of some relief, go ahead, but realize that most experts think it's a lot of effort for nothing.

Cherries and Other Folk Remedies

Not long after Barbara Pollak discovered she had RA, she heard that eating cherries would help, so she gave it a try. "In the spring and summer I would eat cherries constantly. I liked them and I ate them, but I didn't see any big change."

Like Pollak, lots of people with arthritis have wondered about this quaint folk remedy. Some have probably even tried it. Although it's a charming idea, it's not a proven one. According to folklore, cherries are supposed to help relieve gout (*not* RA) by reducing uric acid levels in the blood. But there's no evidence that they actually do that. And even if they did, it wouldn't do much good for Pollak or most other arthritic people. While gout sufferers have a problem with high uric acid, cherries haven't been shown to help them—or anyone else with arthritis.

According to the authors of *Chicken Soup and Other Folk Remedies,* people seeking relief from arthritis should eat up to a dozen cherries a day in addition to drinking a glass of cherry juice. "Find a happy medium by using your own good judgment as to cherry dosage," the authors advise. "Listen to your body. You'll know soon enough if the cherries seem to be making you feel better."

Duck These Dangerous Diets

Thankfully, the list of downright dangerous diets for arthritis is relatively short. Here are the dietary practices you should approach with great caution—or avoid completely.

Fasting. Many elimination diets, which try to identify food sensitivities, start with a fast—you eat no food at all for several days or longer. Unless your fast is supervised by a physician, you run the risk of health problems.

"I don't recommend anyone fasting at home," says Robert M. Stroud, M.D., of the University of Florida College of Medicine. "If people are on various medications, it's especially hazardous." Fasting is a form of stress and is likely to make you weak and tired. More seriously, fasting can upset the balance of minerals and water in your body.

That said, some people with rheumatoid arthritis start to feel better when they fast, although their symptoms return when they eat normally again. This observation, which hasn't been explained yet, may provide researchers with new insights into RA. But for now, it's not of much practical importance. Starving yourself is no way to get better.

Raw food diets. A slice of raw beef liver, anyone? That's one of the supposedly helpful foods recommended in *A Doctor's Proven New Home Cure for Arthritis*. A few other arthritis diets also recommend raw foods, including unpasteurized milk. While natural foods are fine, harmful microorganisms may contaminate unpasteurized milk and other uncooked protein foods and make you sick.

Extremely unbalanced diets. One arthritis diet recommends two to four eggs daily along with at least a quart of milk, a quarter-pound of liver, and lots of meat— virtually the opposite of the low-fat diet advocated elsewhere in this book. Apparently, proponents of this diet want to exchange your arthritis for heart disease. Even if the diet did help your joints, your circulatory system would be drowning in fat and cholesterol. Forget it.

Even if the cherries don't make you feel better, at least they're a nutritious snack: They're virtually fat-free and have small amounts of vitamins A and C. They won't do you any harm— unless you decide to eat cases of cherry pie filling.

The Apple Cider Vinegar Solution

Here's a folk remedy that's much less tasty: Take 1 teaspoon of apple cider vinegar mixed with 1 teaspoon of honey each morning and evening. Or mix 2 ounces of apple cider vinegar with 6 ounces of water. Down the hatch!

The rationale for this home remedy is a little kooky. Supposedly, vinegar thins the body fluids and makes the joints more tender. Honey is said to relieve pain.

"It's true that if you put a piece of meat in vinegar, it will make it more tender—but that's not what happens in your body," says Dr. Wolman. After all, you don't tenderize your innards when you eat oil-and-vinegar dressing, do you? In any event, most people want to make their joints less tender, not more so.

The Potato Trick

Our last folk remedy would have you put food *on* your body rather than *in* it. "Carry a raw potato in your pocket. Don't leave home without it! When it shrivels up after a day or two, replace it with a fresh potato," counsel the authors of *Chicken Soup and Other Folk Remedies*. It sounds like a pitch for the American Express card. Chances for noticeable relief: zero.

PART
3

Move Away from Pain

6

Exercise:
A Perfect Prescription

Ahh, exercise. It probably makes you think of a svelte young woman in an aerobics class, running in place while being serenaded by Michael Jackson. Or perhaps you see a hulking weight lifter, eyes bulging and knees quivering as he struggles to lift a 300-pound barbell.

If you have arthritis, the mere thought of all that huffing, puffing, sweating, and stomping may cause you to look for the nearest easy chair. And that's understandable. When your joints hurt, it's natural to want to coddle them by moving as little as possible. At first, recommending exercise for arthritis may sound about as sensible as telling an insomniac to sleep through a rock concert.

"In this age of the beautiful body, 'they' make exercise look so easy," writes Gwen Ellert, a nurse who has rheumatoid arthritis (RA), in her book *Arthritis and Exercise*. "Just put on your matching shorts, top, and jogging shoes, and head off to exercise class. But it is not as easy it looks. In the morning, I have trouble opening my eyes and getting out of bed on time!"

If that's pretty much how *you* feel about exercise, you're in for some pleasant surprises. First, you don't have to transform yourself into a Jane Fonda or an Arnold Schwarzenegger to reap the benefits of exercise. A gentle, gradual program is all it takes. Second, the right sort of movement may be the *best* thing you can do for your arthritis.

"People with arthritis who exercise can see dramatic results," says champion golfer Jan Stephenson, who stars in an exercise videotape produced by the Arthritis Foundation for people with arthritis. "Exercise can decrease pain and stiffness and may even help [you] to regain function of your joints." Even better, exercise can help you restore your energy and emotional well-being.

Why Doctors Say, "Get Moving!"

Only recently have doctors come to understand how important exercise is for arthritis. For many years, they warned against all but the mildest activity for fear of making arthritis worse. "The old rap was 'The less you exercise, the better off you'll be,' " recalls Bill Warren, an Arizona man who has had osteoarthritis for most of his 69 years. "They forced you into a sedentary life, and they forced on you this attitude of 'Learn to live with it.' "

"I think doctors have missed the boat on exercise," agrees Thomas C. Namey, M.D., a rheumatologist, director of sports medicine, and associate professor of medicine at the University of Tennessee Medical Center in Knoxville. "Doctors have been notorious prescribers of rest. And we've put many people through sedentary lives unnecessarily."

Dr. Namey speaks from personal as well as professional experience. As a young man, he developed psoriatic arthritis, which bothered his knees in particular. A few years later, a skiing accident further injured his right knee. "I thought that was the death knell for me in terms of physical activity," he recalls.

Fortunately, Dr. Namey took his own medical advice and devised an exercise routine for his arthritis. Every morning, he takes a warm shower and limbers up with gentle stretches. In the evenings, he exercises at home by riding his stationary bike or working out on a rowing machine. And on weekends, he's likely to be found bicycling in the nearby countryside with his wife and two children.

Dr. Namey says his fitness program, especially bicycling, has kept his knees virtually pain-free—and forestalled the need for surgery. "Now I have absolutely no pain walking or cycling, unless I really overdo it. Until I was in regular aerobic exercise, I couldn't make that statement.

"If you saw me, you'd have no idea that I have a rheumatic problem," he continues. "I can get on a bike and cycle 100 miles. I couldn't do that when I was 20, but I can do it now—because I'm in better aerobic shape now than when I was 20.

"In a sense, one of the best things that ever happened to me was that I have this arthritis that hurt my knee. It has made me a healthier person all around—and isn't that the most important thing?"

Exercise Soothes Arthritis Seven Ways

If you could discover a pill with as many arthritis-fighting qualities as exercise, you'd be an instant billionaire. Unlike any other medical treatment, exercise battles arthritis on many different fronts at once. Consider what it can do.

It limbers up tight, achy joints. In fact, flexibility is the only antidote to the stiffness that comes with arthritis. And you don't need to huff and puff to improve your flexibility. Gentle stretching or range-of-motion exercises are all that's needed. (These daily exercises, which should be the cornerstone of your fitness plan, are discussed in chapter 7, "Loosening Up: Stretching and Strengthening Exercises.")

It tones your muscles. Strong muscles act like braces around your joints, protecting them from injury. Well-toned muscles also sculpt your figure, something you may have lost through years of "taking it easy."

It is a natural painkiller. Far from causing more pain, a safe, well-designed exercise program makes many people feel *better*. In several studies, arthritis patients who walked, rode stationary bikes, danced, or did pool exercises actually reduced their joint pain and swelling. With regular exercise, some people feel so much better that they need less medication.

It peps you up. If having arthritis makes you feel tired and weak, one reason may be that you're out of shape. Here again, a little exercise goes a long way. One study showed that riding an exercise bike for 15 minutes three times a week boosted the energy levels of people with RA.

It slims you down. More vigorous exercises, such as walking and cycling, are good calorie burners. (See chapter 8, "Moving Forward: Aerobic Exercise.") "Exercise is a wonderful way to lose weight," says Jennifer DePalmer, a Philadelphia woman who has RA. DePalmer, who swims regularly and teaches water aerobics, says the activity has helped her lose 10 pounds. The weight loss, in turn, has kept her back free of pain.

It thickens and strengthens your bones. Exercises such as walking are particularly good because they require you to bear your body weight on your joints. (Swimming and cycling are examples of non-weight-bearing exercises.) Bones respond to this natural stress by absorbing more strength-building calcium. And that calcium provides an added benefit: protection against osteoporosis, the brittle-bone disease that adds to the aches and pains of many people with arthritis.

It boosts your spirits. Vigorous exercise is as good for your mind as your body, says Susan G. Perlman, M.D., a rheumatologist and assistant professor of clinical medicine at Northwestern University School of Medicine in Chicago. Dr. Perlman designed a low-impact dance program specifically for women with RA. She says the women felt empowered by their success at exercise, which gave them the confidence to try new things such as traveling. "They got a real boost to their sense of what they were capable of accomplishing—a sort of can-do attitude," she says. "They felt more optimistic about other options in their lives."

Nursing Joints Back to Health

If a joint stays active, it will do its job with vigor for years. But let a joint sit around doing nothing and before you know it, the whole thing goes to pot. (Come to think of it, joints are a lot like people.)

Consider what happens when a laboratory animal's injured joint is immobilized in a cast for six to ten weeks. Without normal activity, chondrocytes (cells that produce joint cartilage) seem to go to sleep on the job: Their metabolism slows dramatically, and the cartilage itself becomes thin and soft. The neighborhood around the joint—the connective tissue— deteriorates as well. Ligaments and tendons can loosen from their fastenings on the bones, and the muscles shrink and weaken.

But when the cast is removed and exercise is resumed— voilá! —the cartilage is restored to its former condition, and the animal's joint eventually looks normal again. The muscle also returns to normal.

What's the secret of exercise's regenerative powers? In simple terms, nourishment: Without activity, the joint cartilage starves. "Because there is no direct blood supply to the cartilage, all nourishment is by diffusion," explains Dr. Namey. "The way you increase nutrition to the cartilage is by gently squeezing it, like a sponge. Gentle compression and expansion is a way of encouraging diffusion of nutrients into cartilage." Exercise also stimulates ligaments, tendons, and other joint tissues to stay healthy.

But can exercise actually cure or reverse various kinds of arthritis? *Maybe.* A few doctors say exercise is a natural healer for some types of arthritis. John H. Bland, M.D., a University of Vermont College of Medicine rheumatologist, says the right balance of exercise and rest can slow down osteoarthritis and in some rare cases, reverse the disease.

Dr. Bland tells the story of a former patient, an 85-year-old man who was crippled by osteoarthritis of the hips and could hardly get out of bed. Using a cane, and with great effort, the man began a walking program. Before he died at 92, he was walking three-quarters of a mile twice a day. X rays taken before and after he began walking suggest that his arthritic hips had markedly improved.

In Dr. Bland's view, exercise can repair arthritic damage by triggering the chondrocytes to make new cartilage and replacing cartilage worn away by the disease. Dr. Bland emphasizes, though, that exercise has to be carefully balanced with rest and other medical treatments for the repair process to work.

Although many doctors agree with Dr. Bland in theory, they caution that too few studies have been done to confirm his ideas. What *is* certain, says Dr. Namey, is that exercise can help to relieve the *symptoms* of osteoarthritis. "In that sense, exercise is as good as any medication we use for osteoarthritis," he says.

There are also tantalizing hints that exercise may slow the progress of RA. Rolf Nordemar, M.D., a Swedish doctor and a pioneer in the study of exercise and arthritis, came to that conclusion a few years ago after studying 46 patients with RA. Half of the patients exercised daily for a half hour, choosing activities such as swimming, walking, or cycling. The others didn't exercise. After eight years, the exercise group had spent only half as much time in the hospital as the inactive group. But the most important finding came from X rays: When the study ended, the exercise group showed less joint damage than the nonexercisers, suggesting that vigorous activity slowed joint destruction.

Exercise also may prevent fibromyalgia, a painful condition that affects the muscles and other soft tissues around the joints, and help to relieve this condition if you already have it. Studies show that people who exercise regularly are much less likely to get fibromyalgia than sedentary people.

Young Woman Saved by Exercise

Such findings came as no surprise to many people with arthritis. Jennifer DePalmer, for example, knows from first-hand experience what exercise can do. An intelligent, 22-year-old nursing student, she says exercise has kept her RA in remission. And it's hard to doubt her. Slim, athletic, and full of energy, DePalmer looks like she belongs on the cover of a fitness magazine, not in a doctor's office.

But it wasn't always that way. When she learned she had arthritis as a college freshman, she was in bad shape, physically and mentally. Burdened by shooting pains in her wrists and other joints, she sadly abandoned her dream of becoming a professional cellist and decided to become a nurse instead. Fortunately, she found a doctor who told her to stay as active as possible—advice that ultimately restored her health, she believes.

Between nursing school classes, DePalmer swims and gives swimming lessons, teaches water aerobics classes, rides her bike, and walks as much as she can. "I'm sure the exercise I'm doing now is keeping my arthritis under control," she says. "The more I exercise, the fewer flare-ups I have and the less joint problems."

But she didn't fully understand how important exercise was for her until recently. Hospitalized for surgery unrelated to arthritis, Jennifer was bedridden for ten days. To her surprise, the bed rest caused her almost-forgotten arthritis to return with a vengeance, making her knees and ankles burn with pain. "The pain would wake me up in the middle of the night, and I would be in tears," she recalls. "Two or three days later, it dawned on me what had happened. I wasn't getting any exercise and that's what was causing the flare-up."

The next day, she began exercising again in a swimming pool. Because of her recent surgery, she moved gingerly at first, walking in the shallow end and swimming gently. But the mild activity helped. The first night after getting back into the pool, she slept with much less pain. And a few days later, her joint aches had vanished. "It kind of shocked everybody, myself included, because I didn't think exercise could make that kind of difference, much less in the time it took."

DePalmer no longer takes any medication for her RA except for an occasional aspirin. Without exercise, she says, "I would have been in a lot of pain. Getting exercise and being physically active is so essential to me."

Ten Tips to Make Exercise Fun

"What's the difference between play and exercise?" asks Dr. Namey. "It's like the difference between sex and artificial insemination. Both accomplish the same thing, but one is a lot more fun!"

His point: Exercise is most rewarding if it's *play*—if you truly have your heart in it. Your fitness plan should become a lifelong friend you greet with enthusiasm, not feelings of obligation. But what if regular exercise seems about as friendly as a viper? Here are ten tips that can help you turn an exercise grimace into a contented grin.

Give some thought to the kind of exercise you want to do. "Find one type of exercise that you really like, something that, even if you're a little sore the next day, you'll want to go back and do it again," advises DePalmer.

Rekindle the childlike joy of exercise. Think back to

the activities that thrilled you as a child. Maybe you loved to ride your bike or splash around in a backyard pool. Get in touch with those pleasurable feelings.

Chip away at any mental blocks against exercise. Without being aware of it, you may be harboring negative feelings about exercise. Did you sour on exercise when you didn't get picked for the softball team in high school? If you're a woman, did your family laugh at you for being a tomboy? Get rid of unproductive feelings by talking them over with a friend—or looking forward, not backward.

Go for rhythm, not blues. Listen to music with a lively beat while you exercise. Carry a portable radio or cassette player, even if you exercise outside. If you attend a group exercise class, ask your instructor to play your favorite tunes.

Dress for workout success. Give your spirits a lift by buying a new exercise outfit or two in bold, zingy colors. Look for an outfit that's easy to take on and off, such as a pair of pull-on cotton sweatpants with a matching sweatshirt.

Exercise with a buddy. Having a friend to chat with—or just to exchange hard-earned groans—makes time pass quickly and keeps your spirits up.

Join an exercise group. Group classes are a great way to make new friends. Many people also feel more motivated to show up regularly when they're part of a group. If it's a good class, you'll get feedback from the instructor and be able to share your experience with others.

Reward yourself for good behavior. If you stick with your exercise program for a month or so, treat yourself to a new gym bag, a plush terry cloth robe to wear after showering, or even a trial membership in a health club.

Vary your exercise routine. If you're feeling blah about your fitness program, try adding some new exercises or switching to another activity for a while. If you're bored with walking, for example, try walking in a pool. It's fun and a real change of pace.

Don't take exercise too seriously. If you can't do a particular exercise—a leg lift in a low-impact aerobics class, for example—just stop, then jump back in when the class gets to the next activity. Remember, anybody with arthritis who exercises is a trouper. Congratulate yourself for doing your best.

CHAPTER

7

Loosening Up: Stretching and Strengthening Exercises

Carl Williams, who has osteoarthritis in his arms and legs, remembers having too much pain and stiffness to scrub his back in the shower or bend over and pick up a pencil from the floor. And he remembers thinking that he'd have to give up fishing, his favorite hobby, because he could no longer get around easily in his boat.

But Williams fought back with stretching exercises—and won. Since joining an arthritis exercise class at West Jersey Hospital in Evesham, New Jersey, he has regained his former flexibility, and then some. Lean and lithe at 61, Williams now is more limber than most people half his age. "It makes it so I can fish," he exults. "If I hadn't been doing these exercises, I'd be selling my boat about now."

Gwen Ellert, R.N., author of *Arthritis and Exercise,* tells a more dramatic story about what gentle exercise can do. A few years ago, she was an invalid, crippled with severe rheumatoid arthritis (RA). She, too, diligently stuck to a daily program of stretching and strengthening exercises. Now, she walks without a limp and goes out dancing on weekends. "I never could see myself in a wheelchair for the rest of my life," she says. "It just wasn't part of my self-image."

As Williams and Ellert discovered, one of the best ways to outsmart arthritis is to loosen up. But exercises that help you regain strength and flexibility are also the key to your *entire* exercise program: Make them the foundation of your fitness plan, and you'll

soon be moving on to more vigorous activities like swimming or cycling. If you're already active, this chapter will show you how to
gain even greater flexibility and strength.

Getting Set for Exercise

Before you lace up your sneakers and head for the gym, take
a few minutes for a mental exercise—planning. You have to plan
ahead for your new fitness program, just as you would for any other
important change in your life. These six guidelines will help you
launch yourself into fitness.

**Talk to your doctor, and ideally, a physical therapist,
before you start exercising.**   Every case of arthritis is unique,
and you need to know which exercises will work best for you and
which might be harmful. Your doctor may want you to avoid some
movements, especially if you have artificial joints, osteoporosis,
neck or back pain, or have had recent joint surgery. You might
want to take this book along to your next doctor's appointment and
ask which exercises are right for you. (Don't substitute exercises in
this chapter for any that have been prescribed by your doctor or
physical therapist.)

Make exercise a habit.   Set aside a regular time to exercise each day, ideally when you have the least pain and stiffness
(perhaps in the morning after a warm shower). Choose an area of
your home where you won't be distracted and where it's comfortable, warm, and draft-free.

Be patient.   Don't expect instant results—you'll only get
discouraged. Start out slowly, giving your body time to adjust to
your new routine. Gradually do more, always paying attention to
how you feel. Give yourself at least three months before expecting
the exercises to make a real difference in how you feel, suggests
Marilyn Huber, author and developer of ArthroCize, an arthritis
exercise program.

Expect some setbacks, and take them in stride.
"What you can do easily one day, you may not be able to do another day when you're flared up, so you need to adjust your program accordingly," says Susan G. Perlman, M.D., a rheu-

matologist and assistant professor of clinical medicine at North-western University Medical School in Chicago. On days when you do have a flare-up, go easy. Unless your doctor or physical therapist gives you other instructions, try to continue to do some stretching or range-of-motion exercises—even on painful joints and even if all you can manage is a few repetitions.

Don't overdo it. If you go overboard with exercise, you could trigger a flare-up or, worse, rupture a tendon or ligament in an inflamed joint. More likely, you'll just feel so pooped and sore the next day that you'll want to give up. So balance exercise with rest. Expect to feel a little tired after exercise and plan for it, especially if you're just starting out. If you're *totally* worn out after an exercise session, ease up next time. (See the next section for more specific guidelines.)

Think like a winner. "Keep a positive attitude," says Gwen Ellert. "Recognize when you're starting to feel sorry for yourself, and kick yourself out of it." And take pride in what you can accomplish, instead of worrying about what you can't do yet. "If you can do something today that's more than yesterday, that's wonderful," says Wendy McBrair, R.N., an arthritis clinical nurse specialist who has RA.

Pay Attention to Aches and Pains

"We always tell people that the saying, 'no pain, no gain' is strictly for dumb jocks!" laughs Jodi Maron-Barth, a registered physical therapist who is supervisor of physical therapy for arthritis patients at Moss Rehabilitation Hospital in Philadelphia. Arthritis hurts enough as it is. There's no reason for your exercise program to become a pain in the neck—or any other joint. Done correctly, exercise should help you prevent or relieve pain. It should *not* make you feel worse.

"When you finish exercising, you may have some mild discomfort that persists," says Terri Aagaard, M.D., an emergency medicine physician at Pioneer Valley Hospital in Salt Lake City. "But if after an hour your joint is still tender, you've probably overdone it and need to cut back just a little."

Most physical therapists go by the 2-hour pain rule: If your joint still hurts 2 hours after exercise, ease up the next time. Reduce the number of repetitions you do on sensitive joints, or do the same number more gently. "If that doesn't help, pick an alternative exercise that will accomplish the same objective," suggests Huber.

Meanwhile, learn to tune in to and interpret your body's pain messages. You'll discover that not all aches are created equal. For example, sharp or sudden pain that starts during exercise is a danger signal, a warning to change your routine to avoid hurting yourself. Stop doing the exercise immediately, and try a gentler, pain-free version of the movement. If that doesn't help, skip the exercise; there are plenty of others to try.

On the other hand, don't worry about a little muscle soreness, which often develops within a day or two of doing new exercises. Temporary muscle soreness is a sign that unused muscles are adjusting to your new routine. Usually, you can tell the difference between joint pain and muscle soreness by paying close attention to subtle differences in where you hurt. (A certain amount of mild soreness in the "meat" of a muscle— between your elbow and your shoulder or your knee and your hip, for example—is to be expected. Pain in the elbow, shoulder, knee, or hip itself, however, is a sign that something may be wrong. In that case, stop immediately.)

Some Pre-Exercise Tips

Some people find that taking their standard pain-relief medication about 20 minutes before exercise gives the drug a chance to kick in and help prevent undue pain. Dr. Aagaard says that's a good idea but cautions not to take more medicine than normal or use narcotic painkillers like Darvon before or after exercise. She points out that without pain messages to guide you, you might exercise too hard, perhaps causing an injury or damaging a weakened joint. Also, you shouldn't *need* extra pain relief: "Your exercise should not cause pain to the point where you need additional pain medication," she says. "If you're having a lot of pain, then you're not exercising correctly."

The Ice Bag Trick

A better pain-relief tip for exercisers: If you have a hot, swollen joint that you want to exercise gently, try putting an ice pack (wrapped in a towel) on it first. Ellert suggests putting a bag of frozen peas on the joint for about 10 minutes before you exercise. When you're done, put the bag into the freezer to use another day. Don't keep ice on your joint for more than about 20 minutes, however, or the pain may return. Using ice is an exception to the general rule that it's best to warm up before exercise. Save this tip for badly flared joints, and use it *sparingly*.

The Warm-Up

Remember playing with Turkish taffy as a kid? On a warm day, the taffy was soft and stretchable. But if the temperature dipped, the taffy became brittle and cracked easily. In the same way, your muscles stretch more easily if you warm up before exercise, and may tear if you don't, says Sharon Foy, director of the International Exer-Safety Association, a Cleveland organization devoted to promoting safe exercise.

Warming up stimulates blood flow to your muscles, making them relaxed and easier to move. In the past, warm-up routines usually were stretching exercises, says Marilyn Huber. Now fitness experts say you should literally make your body warm before you begin any stretching. The following warm-up methods can do the job.

● March or walk in place slowly for 5 minutes or so, until you feel your body giving off some heat. Swing your arms, if you can, but not above shoulder level. If you need support, hold on to the back of a chair.

● If you don't walk easily, a warm shower or soak in a bathtub for 15 or 20 minutes can warm muscles.

● A hot water bottle or heating pad can warm joints you want to exercise. (But remember, avoid heat if joints are badly inflamed and swollen.)

- Stand a comfortable distance in front of a radiator or space heater until the parts of your body you want to exercise feel relaxed and warm.
- Massage can help, too. With the palm of your hand, rub the muscles around the joint in a gentle circling motion, but don't rub the joint itself.

As part of your warm-up routine, spend a few minutes practicing breathing exercises. They'll help you tune into your body and will bring more nourishing oxygen to every cell. Here's the breathing exercise that Huber uses in her ArthroCize classes in South Bend, Indiana.

Sit comfortably in a chair with both feet on the floor. With your shoulders relaxed and both hands on your abdomen, slowly inhale through your nose. You should feel your abdomen start to expand like a balloon. Next, exhale through your mouth, making a "shhh" or "ahhh" sound. "Try to focus on breathing deeper than your normal everyday pattern," says Huber. Breathe slowly and rhythmically. Do this breathing exercise three times, then return to your normal breathing pattern.

A final reminder: Don't hold your breath when you exercise. While it's a natural tendency to hold your breath when you're really exerting yourself, it can raise blood pressure and starve muscles of oxygen. If you find yourself holding your breath, focus on your breathing and say "ahhh" as you exhale for several breaths. Or try singing or counting out loud, which makes holding your breath impossible.

Ready, Set, Stretch

Once you're warmed up, you're ready to begin stretching. (See "Stretching Exercises" on page 92 for instructions on specific stretches.) Think of yourself as a graceful ballet dancer. "Stretching movements should be slow and gentle," says Huber. "There should never be any fast, jerky movements." Above all, never stretch with a bouncing motion, which may tear muscle fibers.

(continued on page 97)

Stretching Exercises

You can do the following exercises either sitting or standing. (If you're in a wheelchair, check first with your doctor or physical therapist for variations that might be right for you.)

If you like, you can do the exercises while listening to music or watching television. Gwen Ellert, R.N., advises people to try between three and ten repetitions for each exercise, and fewer if you have a hot, swollen joint. For joints that don't have arthritis or no longer bother you, ten repetitions may be no problem.

Don't worry if you can't do a particular exercise—skip it and go on to the next one. You may also want to show these illustrations to your doctor, who can advise you if any of these exercises aren't appropriate for you. Your doctor's go-ahead is especially important if you have any artificial joints.

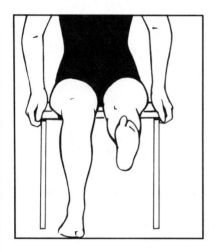

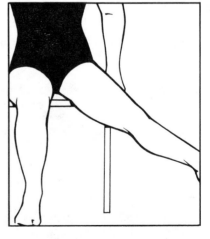

Spreadeagles. Here's a leg exercise that can be helpful if you have trouble getting into a bathtub or in and out of your car. While seated in a chair, straighten one leg in front of you, with your foot raised slightly. Slowly move your leg to the side, then bring it back to the center. Relax. Repeat with the other leg. (Check with your doctor before doing this exercise if you've had hip surgery.)

Note: Some of these exercises were adapted from the Arthritis Foundation Exercise Program, with permission. Others were developed in consultation with Jodi Maron-Barth, a physical therapist at the Moss Rehabilitation Hospital, Philadelphia.

Head tilts. Seated or standing, with your shoulders relaxed, tilt your head to the right, moving the right ear over the right shoulder. Slowly return to center, then tilt toward your left shoulder. Continue to look forward as you move.

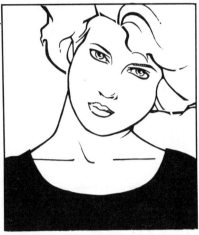

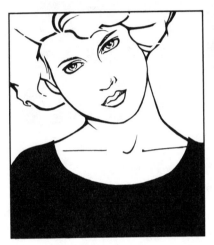

Back scratcher. This exercise may help if you have trouble zipping a dress or washing your back in the shower. Seated or standing, roll up a kitchen towel or dishcloth and hold it in your right hand. Bring the towel up over your right shoulder and let it drop down your back. Grab the lower end with your left hand. Then give yourself a slow back rub, pulling the towel back and forth. Gently lift your lower arm as you pull the towel up. (Check with your doctor before doing this exercise if you've had shoulder surgery.)

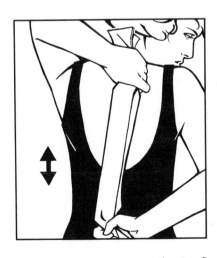

(continued)

Stretching Exercises—*Continued*

Shoulder circles. Seated or standing, slowly circle both of your shoulders, lifting them up, then forward, down and back. Repeat in the opposite direction.

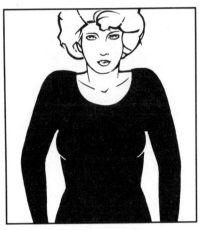

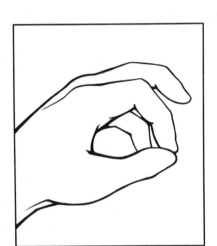

Hand O's. This exercise may help if you have trouble grasping pencils, silverware, and other small objects. Touch the tip of your thumb to the tip of your index finger, making a perfect *O* shape. Separate and straighten your fingers. Repeat, using your thumb with each of your other fingers. (Check with your doctor about doing this exercise if you've had hand or wrist surgery.)

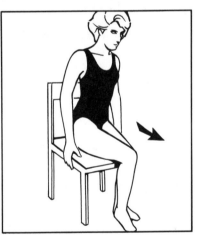

Hip walk. "Walking" to the front edge of your chair and back again can help keep your hips flexible. For each step, lift one buttock and move it forward, then lift the other buttock and advance.

Beach ball swings. While seated, carry the ball across your body, all the way from your right side to your left. Keep your arms extended at about shoulder height. (Check with your doctor before doing this exercise if you've had shoulder surgery.)

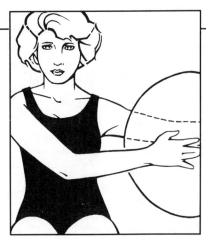

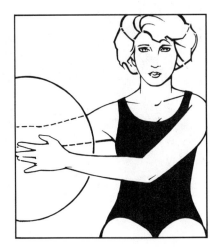

Balloon bounces. To keep your arms and shoulders flexible, try keeping a balloon aloft with one arm at a time. Standing, with your palm facing up, hit the balloon upward, and try to keep it in the air as you raise and lower your arm. (Check with your doctor before doing this exercise if you've had elbow or shoulder surgery.)

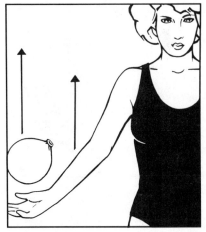

(continued)

Stretching Exercises—*Continued*

Calf stretches. This is a good warm-up exercise to do before walking. Stand and put your hands on a chair or table for support, if you need it. Bend one knee slightly and put the other leg behind you, keeping both feet flat on the floor. Lean forward, with your back knee straight. Feel the stretch in your back calf? If not, step back a little farther. Hold the stretch for a count of ten and relax. Repeat with the other leg.

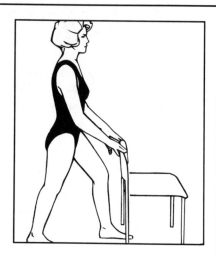

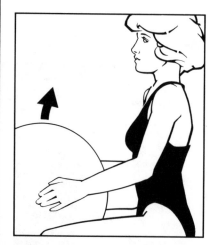

Beach ball lifts. While seated, slowly lift a beach ball from your knees over your head, then lower again. Look forward as you lift, and don't tilt your head back. Use a light couch pillow if you don't have a ball. (Check with your doctor before doing this exercise if you've had shoulder surgery.)

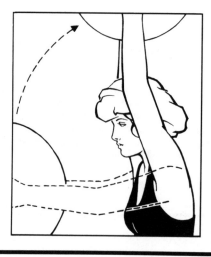

Move each joint just to the point of discomfort, then stop. It's usually safe to push slightly beyond the first hint of discomfort, but never go to the point of causing sharp pain.

Sometimes, people with severe arthritis need the help of a physical therapist to do a particular exercise. However, never let anyone else assist you with stretching exercises by pushing or pulling; you could push a joint past its safety zone.

The Next Step: Strengthening Exercises

Once you can stretch comfortably, you may be able to add some muscle-toning exercises to your routine. Fortunately, you don't need to bulk up or become a power lifter to build stronger muscles. In fact, most physical therapists advise against working out with weights, which may overstress weakened joints. A better idea: isometric exercises, which are easier to do and put much less strain on joints because they tighten and hold the muscle without moving joints. An example of an isometric exercise is pressing your hands together and holding for 6 seconds. If you do the exercise regularly, just those few seconds of contraction are enough to strengthen the muscle. (See "Strengthening Exercises" on page 98 for examples of this type of exercise.)

As your muscles get stronger, you can have fun and get a more challenging workout with rubber exercise bands, available in many retail stores. To use a band, wrap it around your legs, either a few inches above your knees or above your ankles, and tie the ends together. (Or you can loop one end around your ankle and the other around a chair leg.) The idea is to walk and step out to the side or forward with one leg, all of which provides resistance and tones your muscles. The higher you wear the band—that is, the closer to your torso—the greater the resistance it provides. Conversely, wearing the band just above your ankles provides less resistance. The next section shows several exercises you can do with or without the bands.

A few cautions: Don't try an exercise with a band until you can easily do the same exercise without it. To use a band safely, always

(continued on page 100)

Strengthening Exercises

If you're just starting out, try to do each of these exercises two or three times. Gradually increase the number of repetitions to ten. (If you have hypertension or heart disease, check with your doctor before doing isometric exercises, since they can cause temporary increases in blood pressure.)

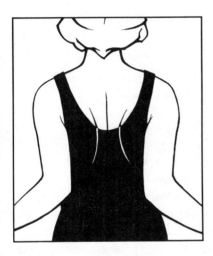

Shoulder blade pinches. Seated or standing, try to pinch your shoulder blades together by moving your shoulders and elbows as far back as possible. Hold for a count of five and relax.

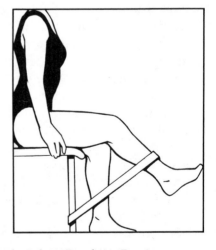

Leg lifts plus. For a greater challenge, loop an exercise band under your chair leg and slip your foot through the other end. Keep the loop a few inches above your ankle. Try to straighten your knee until the band is tight. Hold for a count of five and relax. (Check with your doctor about doing this exercise if you've had knee surgery.)

Note: Some of these exercises were adapted from the Arthritis Foundation Exercise Program, with permission. Others were developed in consultation with Jodi Maron-Barth, a physical therapist at the Moss Rehabilitation Hospital, Philadelphia.

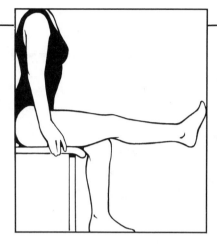

Leg lifts. This knee-strengthening exercise and the following one can help you climb stairs and get in and out of chairs. While seated, slowly raise one foot to straighten your leg; hold for a count of five, then bring it down again. Alternate your right and left leg. (Check with your doctor about doing this exercise if you've had knee surgery.)

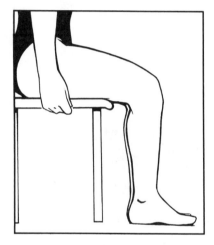

Tummy toners. Try this exercise for a flatter stomach. Sit in a chair with an upright back, keeping the small of your back touching the chair. Lift both feet off the floor, holding the seat of the chair for support. Hold for five counts and relax. Keep breathing. You should feel this exercise in your lower abdominal muscles. (Check with your doctor before doing these exercises if you've had hip or knee surgery.)

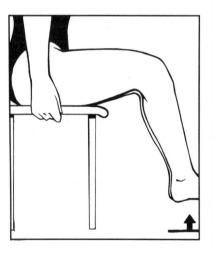

(continued)

Strengthening Exercises—*Continued*

A

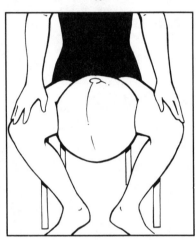

B

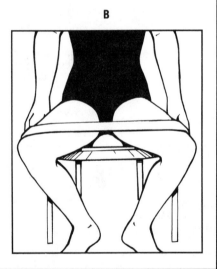

Thigh toners. (A) While seated, squeeze a beach ball between your knees. Hold for a count of five and release. (B) Also while seated, loop an exercise band around your thighs, a few inches above your knees. Spread your knees apart until you feel the resistance. Hold for a count of five and relax. (Check with your doctor before doing this exercise if you've had hip surgery.)

loop it a few inches above a joint, never on the joint itself. People with troublesome knees should tie bands only *above* the knees to prevent undue strain on the knees. Also, don't use the band if your joints are swollen or if it causes any pain. And one final caution: People with hypertension also should be careful about using high-resistance bands, which can temporarily raise blood pressure.

Dyna-Band Total Body Toners are commercially available exercise bands, color-coded according to how much resistance they provide. The pink ones have the least resistance and the green ones medium resistance. If you can't locate Dyna-Bands in stores in your area, you can order them by mail by writing to Fitness Wholesale, Inc., 3064 West Edgerton Road, Silver Lake, OH 44224, or call 1-800-537-5512.

To make your own exercise bands, simply cut the elastic waistband from a pair of men's boxer shorts, suggests Jodi Maron-Barth. If you need a longer band, cut two waistbands and sew them together.

The Cool-Down

When you finish exercising, you may feel like plopping down onto the couch. Don't. Take about 5 minutes to gradually slow down and unwind. This cool-down period lets your heart rate return to normal and gives you a chance to relax away the tension of exercise.

To cool down, gradually slow the pace of whatever activity you've been doing for 1 minute. Then, either standing or sitting, take a few deep breaths, reaching your arms up toward the ceiling as you inhale. Bring your arms back down as you exhale, quietly saying "shh."

As you relax further, close your eyes and concentrate on your inner body. "Go through your whole body and review your muscles," says Marilyn Huber. "If there's some area of tension or tightness, focus on that general area and tell it to relax." See if you can picture what the pain or tension looks like, then imagine yourself melting, dissolving, or pushing it away. Spend a few moments enjoying the quiet, and congratulate yourself for doing something wonderful for yourself. Then open your eyes. You're done!

Put an *X* through These Exercises

While many stretching and strengthening exercises are terrific for people with arthritis, a few are dangerous. Although the exercises we're about to describe are potentially harmful for everybody, they're double trouble for people with joint problems, says Sharon

Foy of the International Exer-Safety Association. Here's what to avoid.

Full sit-ups. This is the old-fashioned way of doing a sit-up. With this exercise, you lie down, usually with both legs extended straight out, and try to sit up as far as you can, This exercise, intended to tone abdominal muscles, is torture for your lower back. Curl-ups are a safer alternative: Lie on your back with your knees bent and your lower back pressed into the floor. With your hands loosely clasped behind your head, curl up slightly by raising your shoulders a few inches off the floor. Lie back down. (As an alternative, do this with your arms outstretched in front of you instead of clasped behind your head.)

Double leg raises. This exercise, which is even more dangerous for the lower back than full sit-ups, calls for you to raise both legs off the ground at once while lying on your back. How to do this one safely? You can't, says Foy. If you want to tone your abdominal muscles (the supposed benefit of double leg raises), do the curl-ups described above.

Deep knee bends. Squatting exercises can overstretch the ligaments in your knees, making them unstable, says Foy. They also strain the knees if done in an unstable position, says one doctor. To do this exercise safely, don't bend down beyond the point where your heels begin to lift off the floor. If you have arthritis in your lower body, however, you may want to skip knee bends altogether.

Toe touches. Bending over to touch your toes also can strain your lower back. Get the same flexibility benefits by lying on your back with both knees bent. Then lift one knee and bring it to your chest, pulling it gently toward you with your hands. (Grasp your leg above or below the knee, not on the knee itself.) Repeat with the other knee.

Fire hydrants. In this exercise, you make like a four-legged animal, resting your weight on your hands and knees. Then keeping your right (or left) leg bent at the knee, you lift your other leg out to the side. This is murder on your hips and lower back, says Foy. People with RA also find it hurts their hands. Jane Fonda calls this exercise "Rover's Revenge," and rightly so: It's better left to the dogs.

Exercises "To Go"

Too busy or tired to exercise? Some evenings, so is Wendy McBrair, who works as an arthritis clinical nurse specialist at West Jersey Hospital. But McBrair, who also has RA, has found an ingenious way to fit exercise into her hectic schedule.

"I do a lot of range-of-motion exercises and isometrics at weird times. People don't even know I'm doing them," she says, smiling. It's hard to catch her in the act, but she frequently does ankle circles at meetings, fanny pinches on the phone, and knee exercises while watching television. "I'm probably better about doing those little things than the regular exercise program," she says. "My lifestyle is such that when I get home, I'm tired, and I don't always feel like doing a half-hour exercise program."

Does this mean that taking out the garbage or lifting a half gallon of ice cream qualifies as exercise? Unfortunately, no. Try to stick to your regular exercise routine for the greatest benefits. But when you're especially busy, you can do *some* of your regular exercises at irregular times. Here are some suggestions to get you going, but you can make up others.

In meetings. If you're seated at a table, no one will know if you decide to do some ankle exercises. Here's how: Extend one leg slightly and make a small circling motion with your foot. Circle clockwise a few times, then go counterclockwise. Repeat with the other leg. Or use your pointed foot to draw numbers in the air, from one to ten. Then switch to the other leg.

On the phone. Try some fanny pinches. Tighten your buttocks together and hold for a count of five. Relax and repeat. Or do some toe curls: Slip off your shoes and try to pick up a pencil with your toes. You don't need to actually lift the pencil to experience the benefit.

Watching television. Leg lifts can strengthen your quadriceps, the large muscle in the front of your thigh. Sitting in your favorite chair, slowly raise one foot up until your leg is straight. Hold straight for 3 seconds, then relax. Repeat with the other leg. An alternative exercise: Put your feet up on a footstool. Tighten your thigh for 6 seconds by pressing your knee downward. Repeat several times for each leg.

Washing dishes. When your hands are relaxed in the warm water, spread your fingers apart as far as you can, then bring them back together again. Or gently curl your fingers into a loose fist, then fan your fingers apart to straighten them.

Standing in line. Try shoulder shrugs. Raise your left shoulder toward your ear and lower it again. Then raise the right shoulder, first making sure the left shoulder is relaxed and lowered all the way.

How to Find an Arthritis Exercise Class

Want to share a meaningful smile—or heartfelt groan—with others while you exercise? Consider joining an arthritis exercise class. "I'd recommend a group," says Carl Williams, who attends such a program at West Jersey Hospital. "It makes you feel better about doing the exercises. It's more fun and less labor."

Besides meeting new people, you'll get feedback from the instructor about what you're doing right or wrong. And as you make friends in the class, you may find yourself—surprise!—actually looking forward to exercise. Another plus: Unlike exercise leaders in most health clubs, your instructor is likely to be trained to teach people with arthritis.

In the class Williams attends, the participants sit in a circle on chairs while a physical therapist leads them through stretching and strengthening exercises for half an hour. Afterward, most of the people in the class stay to chat and drink juice.

If you're interested in joining a similar class, call your local chapter of the Arthritis Foundation. The organization's national office has developed an exercise program called PACE, an acronym for People with Arthritis Can Exercise. PACE programs are offered by many local chapters nationwide. Most chapters also offer a water exercise program. (See chapter 9, "Catch the Wave: Aquatic Exercise.")

A number of hospitals and community centers have arthritis exercise classes too, and your chapter of the Arthritis Foundation may know if outside programs are available in your community. If not, check with your physical therapist or rheumatologist. Also call nearby arthritis centers, which are usually affiliated with hospitals, to see if they have an arthritis exercise class open to the public.

Another alternative is to hold an arthritis exercise class right in your own home, with the help of one of several videotapes. Invite a friend over for your video workout, or coax your spouse to exercise with you. Here's what's available.

PACE videotapes, Levels 1 and 2. The Arthritis Foundation's gentle exercise programs are led by champion golfer Jan Stephenson, who is also an exercise consultant. The Level 1 program, which can be done sitting or standing, includes exercises to improve flexibility, strengthen muscles, and increase endurance. The Level 2 program, which is longer and faster paced, is a more challenging workout that includes floor exercises. To order, write: Arthritis Foundation PACE Order Center, 1800 Robert Fulton Drive, Reston, VA 22091.

***Jane Powell's Fight Back with Fitness* videotape (Karl-Lorimar Home Video).** The movie actress leads a group of people who have arthritis—not models—through 25 minutes of warm-ups and 22 minutes of floor exercises. Like the PACE tape, the exercises are designed mainly to improve flexibility and strength. Some of the floor exercises may be difficult for people with severe arthritis or artificial joints, and we recommend you get your doctor's okay before you start. (If he isn't familiar with this tape, you might be better off starting with the PACE tape.) If the Jane Powell tape is not available at your video store, ask about ordering it.

The ROM Dance Program. This relaxing routine is based on the ancient Chinese exercise T'ai Chi Ch'uan, which emphasizes graceful, flowing movements. ROM, developed at St. Marys Hospital Medical Center in Madison, Wisconsin, stands for range of motion, and the program is available as videotapes, a pair of audiocassettes, or an illustrated book. For prices and ordering information, write to the ROM Institute, New Ventures of Wisconsin, Inc., 3601 Memorial Drive, Madison, WI 53704, or call (608) 249-6670.

8

Moving Forward:
Aerobic Exercise

Remember how much fun you had riding your bike when you were a kid, or hiking through the woods, or breaking into an impromptu dance when you heard your favorite song?

Well, it's time to let the child in you come out and play. Walking, bicycling, and dancing—any moderate exertion that makes your heart work a little harder—can be as much fun to do now as when you were nine. In fact, aerobic exercise can almost make you feel like you're nine again. Consider these findings.

● At the University of Missouri Multipurpose Arthritis Center, a group of people with rheumatoid arthritis (RA) and osteoarthritis walked their way to better health. After 12 weeks of walking three times a week, the exercisers had less joint pain and swelling, and their hearts were in better shape.

● At the University of Michigan Medical School, women with RA pedaled away fatigue and stiffness on exercise bicycles. As little as 15 minutes of exercise three times a week was enough to improve fitness in some people.

● In Chicago, women with RA worked out in a modified low-impact aerobic dance program. After 16 weeks, researchers found the women had more endurance, greater energy, and less depression.

Can people with arthritis exercise strenuously enough to improve fitness without aggravating their disease? The answer is yes, says Marian Minor, a physical therapist and a clinical instructor at the University of Missouri School of Medicine, Columbia, and key investigator in the walking study. Aerobic exercise strengthens the most important muscle in your body: your heart. It improves your overall fitness, banishing the fatigue that so often comes with arthritis. And with more energy, you'll get out and about and do more things.

Even better, aerobic exercise appears to soothe painful, swollen joints in some people. Among those who joined the low-impact dancing program, for example, almost all of those who exercised at least twice a week had fewer tender, swollen joints, says Paul Caldron, D.O., a rheumatologist at the Arthritis Center in Phoenix, Arizona, and one of the study's investigators. In some cases, the improvement was dramatic.

Scientists haven't figured out how aerobic exercise soothes painful joints, but Dr. Caldron speculates that endorphins, the body's natural analgesic system, may be involved. In addition, improved blood flow to the joints may cool down local inflammation, he adds. Although the pain-relieving effects of aerobic exercise have been shown in several studies, more research is needed to confirm and understand these exciting findings, he says.

Meanwhile, doctors are encouraging most patients with arthritis to get moving in an aerobic exercise program. This chapter will show you how to start, with a choice of activities that are fun, effective, and—most important for people with sensitive joints—safe.

Aerobics for Beginners

What kind of aerobic exercise should you do? There is no one-size-fits-all answer. Many people with arthritis in their backs or legs wouldn't dream of jogging. But if you have osteoarthritis only in your hands, you probably could run. Similarly, not everyone should exercise at the same intensity. "There is no one level of exercise," says Minor. "It all depends on the individual."

To qualify as aerobic, exercise must meet two simple criteria: It must raise your heart rate, and it must burn oxygen. Activities that use the large muscles—arms or legs or both—and keep you moving for at least 20 to 30 minutes do just that. So a brisk walk around the block may be just as aerobic as jumping rope—without huffing and puffing or sweating and straining. Swimming, bicycling, or dancing also fill the bill. Even gardening can be considered aerobic if you're weeding, spading, and doing other energetic chores around the yard.

To find the right aerobic exercise for you, select an activity that fits your lifestyle and physical condition. The following four steps will help you figure out what kind and how much exercise to do.

Experiment with different types of aerobic exercise until you find something you like. "Perhaps arthritis prevents you from doing your old exercise activities as well as you used to," says Thomas C. Namey, M.D., a rheumatologist, director of sports medicine, and associate professor of medicine at the University of Tennessee Medical Center in Knoxville. "But you can find other things to do, and perhaps do them better than you thought. Think of this 'shopping around' for exercise as you would any other shopping venture. You might not like the first thing you encounter, but if you try three or four activities, you're bound to find something you enjoy."

Get back into shape gradually. For some people, 5 minutes of cycling or walking is plenty for the first few sessions. Each week, try to increase your workout a bit. To find out whether you're exerting yourself sufficiently without working too hard, take your pulse and compare it to the target heart rate for your age. (For directions, see "Finding Your Target Heart Rate" on page 110.)

Synchronize your exercise routine to the natural ups and downs of arthritis pain. If you're having a really bad day, don't do anything strenuous until you feel better. However, don't let a mild flare-up stop you from exercising altogether, says Dr. Caldron. Just exercise for as long as you can manage, as intensely as is comfortable for you.

Consult with your doctor about what kinds of aerobic exercise suit you best. Some people who have badly damaged joints can do aerobic exercise only after undergoing joint replacement surgery and rehabilitation. It's also a good idea to check with your doctor if you haven't exercised recently or are at risk for heart disease.

Getting the go-ahead from your doctor before starting to exercise will give you confidence. Nevertheless, you should stop exercising right away and see your doctor if you become severely short of breath, dizzy, or sick to your stomach, or if you feel pain or tightness in your chest, arm, or throat.

Walking: Steps in the Right Direction

Okay, so maybe you weren't born to run—or play squash or do jumping jacks, for that matter. But with a good pair of shoes, many people with arthritis can *walk* their way to fitness.

While walking is good exercise for everyone, it's especially beneficial for many people with arthritis. Walking is much less jarring than running. Runners hit the pavement with three times the force of their body weight on their joints. But when you walk, the force on your joints is not much more than your own body weight.

Lorraine Lamport of Spencer, Iowa, is among those with arthritis who benefit from regular walks. Lamport, who has osteoarthritis in her knees, started walking for fitness about seven years ago, and now she walks 2 or 3 miles several times a week, often at dawn. "The sunrise in the morning is just beautiful. I walk down past the river on a street with no houses. Once in a while, I'll see a deer. It's very pleasant." The exercise helps her sleep better, gives her more energy, and seems to help her knees. "I've noticed that when my knees are bothering me, walking seems to relieve some of the soreness," she says.

The Greek physician Hippocrates once said, "Walking is man's best medicine." And many present-day doctors would agree. "I think walking is a fantastic exercise," says Dr. Namey. "It can be done at any clip, up or down an incline, indoors or out. If you walk outdoors, the psychological benefits are tremendous."

Walking isn't for everyone with arthritis, though. People with severe arthritis in their hips, knees, ankles, or feet may find any

(continued on page 112)

Finding Your Target Heart Rate

To get the most out of aerobic exercise, you've got to put your heart into it. Whether you cycle, walk, or weed your garden, the exercise should be strenuous enough to push your heart rate into its "target" or "training" range. Aerobic exercise should make your heart pump faster than it does at rest, in a range that will condition the muscle to become stronger and more efficient.

To measure your heart rate, count your pulse for 6 seconds and add a zero. If you count 10 beats in 6 seconds, for example, your heart rate is 100 beats per minute.

The Arthritis Foundation offers these guidelines for finding your pulse: To find your wrist pulse, hold your arm with your palm facing you. Put the index and middle fingers of your other hand on the center of your wrist. Slide your fingertips toward the outside (thumb side) of your wrist and down over two tendons and into a soft depression between the tendons and the bone on the thumb side of your wrist. Apply gentle pressure in that depression and try to feel your pulse. (Your pulse may be more prominent—and easier to measure—on one wrist than on the other.)

Some people have better luck taking the carotid artery pulse in their neck. To find it, put your fingers behind your earlobe and slide them straight down below your jawline. To feel the pulse in the artery, apply gentle pressure.

Your target heart rate is based on your age. You can estimate it from the accompanying table, which gives target heart rates for ages in five-year increments, or you can figure out your range for your actual age. First find your age-adjusted maximum heart rate by subtracting your age from 220 beats per minute. Exercising at this rate is too strenuous and tiring to strengthen your heart. Most exercise experts say that you should try to exercise at 60 to 75 percent of the maximum rate—the "target" heart rate.

If you are 52, for example, your maximum heart rate would be 220 minus 52, or 168 beats per minute. Your target heart rate range would be between 60 percent of 168 (which is 101) and 75 percent of 168 (which is 126). Thus, your heart should be pumping between 101 and 126 beats per minute to get a training effect from exercise.

If you're out of shape, start with no more than 5 to 10 minutes of aerobic exercise and gear your activity to the lower part of your target zone. As your stamina improves, you may gradually build up to a 30-minute workout and aim toward the higher level of your target zone.

Take your pulse before you exercise and every 5 minutes or so during the aerobic activity, suggests Thomas C. Namey, M.D., of the University of Tennessee Medical Center. Use your target heart rate to pace your exercise program, speeding up or slowing down to stay within the right level of exertion. After you stop exercising, your pulse should return to its resting level within half an hour. If it's still high, you've overdone it; cut back a little next time.

Age	Target Heart Rate (60 to 75% of age-predicted maximum, in beats per minute)	10-Second Count
20	120–150	20–25
25	117–146	19–24
30	114–143	19–24
35	111–139	18–23
40	108–135	18–23
45	105–131	17–22
50	102–128	17–21
55	99–124	16–21
60	96–120	16–20
65	93–116	15–19
70	90–113	15–19
75	87–109	14–18
80	84–105	14–18
85	81–101	13–17
90	78–98	13–16

SOURCE: Arthritis Foundation, instructor's manual for the PACE (People with Arthritis Can Exercise) Program.

kind of weight-bearing exercise, including walking, too painful. For those people, water exercises (described in chapter 9, "Catch the Wave: Aquatic Exercise") may be a better alternative.

How can you tell if walking is right for you? "If you can stand and walk comfortably during daily activities, you can probably walk for fitness," says Linda Bocchichio, D.C., a chiropractor in St. James, Long Island, and founder of the St. James Walking Club.

If you enjoy walking and find time to walk often, you'll do your whole body a favor. Consider these benefits.

• Walking can toughen up your bones. Because walking is a weight-bearing exercise, your bones respond by absorbing more calcium, a mineral that thickens and strengthens your skeleton. So walking helps to guard against osteoporosis, the fragile bone disease that plagues many people with arthritis (as well as many others, just due to age).

• Walking can lessen the burden on your joints, because the exercise will result in weight loss. Besides burning up calories, walking helps to control your appetite.

• Walking is an effective way to strengthen your heart. In a study at Stanford University, researchers found that the rate of heart attack for people who walked as few as five city blocks or climbed five flights of stairs daily was lower than the average rate. The more they walked, the greater the benefits. The researchers concluded that people could significantly improve their heart health by walking 9 miles a week.

• Walking is a natural mood elevator. "It makes you feel more alert and energetic," says Gus Fantine, a Long Island resident who belongs to Dr. Bocchichio's outdoor walking club. "You might think after walking, I'd just feel like collapsing, but that's not the case. Walking gears me up to do *more*."

Starting a Walking Program

So, if your doctor or a friend tells you to "take a walk," don't be offended! It's excellent advice. Here are some guidelines to get started.

Buy yourself a pair of thickly cushioned, properly fitting walking shoes. (For tips, see "Finding Fitness Shoes That Fit" on page 122.) A pair of Sorbothane inserts (shock-absorbing inner soles that are sold in many stores specializing in athletic shoes) can add extra cushioning.

Walk on a resilient surface. Look for a relatively soft, level, smooth surface, such as a well-maintained dirt path, an outdoor running track, a golf course after hours, or the wooden floor in a gymnasium. These surfaces have more give than concrete or pavement, making them easier for people with arthritis to walk on. If you do walk on concrete sidewalks or roads, it's essential to wear well-cushioned shoes. For beginning walkers, flat surfaces are easier than hills.

Plan to walk regularly—ideally, three or four times a week. "Get into a routine so it becomes part of your life, not something you do now and then," advises Dr. Bocchichio. "Set aside a time of day for yourself to walk."

Begin with a warm-up. Walk slowly for a few minutes to warm your muscles and increase your heart rate, then do some gentle stretching to loosen your muscles and tendons. Calf stretches are good, but don't forget to stretch your neck, shoulders, and torso, too. (See chapter 7, "Loosening Up: Stretching and Strengthening Exercises.")

Increase your pace and distance gradually. If you walk just halfway around the track your first time, that's fine. After all, you're not competing in a track and field event! Each time you walk, go a little bit farther. You might keep a log of how far you walk each day, how long you walk, and how you feel afterward. "Ideally, you want to build up to walking 45 minutes to an hour," says Dr. Bocchichio. Other experts say 30 to 40 minutes is a reasonable goal.

Walk at a pace that lets you breathe easily. "You should be able to hold a normal conversation without getting out of breath," says Dr. Bocchichio. If you can't talk because you're huffing and puffing too hard, slow down until you can talk.

Practice good walking form. Let your arms swing naturally as you walk, which will help to tone your upper body and make the exercise more aerobic. Correct walking consists of a natural rocking motion: You land first on your heel, then roll toward your toes and push off. Keep your feet pointed straight ahead.

Cool down. During the last 5 or 10 minutes of your walk, slow down, so your heart can gradually return to its resting rate. When you do stop, spend a little time stretching again, which will help to prevent muscle soreness the following day, says Dr. Bocchichio.

Ten Ways to Take a Walk

Give it some thought, and you'll discover plenty of suitable places to walk in your area. Here are ten ideas.

Walk the mall. Many shopping malls welcome walkers and open their doors a few hours early to cater to foot traffic in their corridors. Walking in a mall is great if the weather is nasty or if noisy traffic or outdoor pollutants bother you. Some malls distribute diagrams showing the distances from point to point so you can keep track of your mileage.

Explore your community on foot. You might be amazed at what you discover about your own neighborhood. Sniff the aromas from a local bakery, investigate yard sales, or take in the sights of a street fair. If you're looking for new places to visit, check your community newspaper for local events and attractions.

Take a nature walk. Explore some of the trails in local parks or along lakes, rivers, or canals. Or take a drive to a botanical garden or arboretum and stroll through the grounds. To get the most from your treks, take along binoculars, a camera, or field guides to help you identify birds, trees, and flowers.

Walk to work. If your office is relatively close, use your feet for transportation and forget about traffic and parking hassles. If your workplace is out of walking range, you can park a few blocks from your job site or, if you take public transportation, get off a stop or two ahead of time.

Take a "walking break" instead of a coffee break. The change of pace—and scenery—will refresh you and help you refocus your energy for the rest of the day.

Don't run an errand when you can walk one instead. Next

Pedaling Power

Looking for a year-round fitness activity? Nothing beats a stationary bicycle, which you can pedal in comfort in any season. On an exercise bike, you can strengthen your heart and lungs without fear of hitting a pothole, taking a spill, or dodging speed demons in sports cars.

---

time you're about to drive to the bank or the video store, consider walking instead. If you plan to carry groceries or other packages back with you, wear a backpack or take a collapsible shopping cart with you. (Don't carry heavy items in your arms; this can strain your back.)

Take a walking holiday. There's a walking vacation for just about every travel destination. You can walk from one charming Vermont country inn to the next, for example, while a van ferries your luggage for you. Your travel agent can provide you with information on other walking vacations. Or you can gather brochures and guidebooks and dream up your own itineraries.

Join a walking club. Many communities have walking clubs that sponsor special outings and provide information to members. If your area doesn't have a walking club, get four or five people together and start your own.

Sign up for a walking event. Many nonprofit organizations hold annual walkathons, where people get together to walk for a good cause. Or you can walk in the wake of local jogging races, as Long Island's St. James Walking Club sometimes does. Check your local newspaper for notices of walking events in your community.

Walk your dog. A well-trained dog makes a good companion for solitary walkers and provides a sense of security. If your dog turns walking into a game of tug-of-war with the leash, enroll your pooch in a dog obedience course to teach him or her to heel. (This is important because hard tugging can injure your wrist or hand.) Alternatively, some cats can also be persuaded to walk at the end of a leash.

Pedaling an exercise bike is an excellent aerobic activity if you have arthritis. Riding a bicycle does not require that your feet, ankles, knees, and hips support your body weight. The bicycle seat does it all, and there's minimal stress on joints. "Cycling is an ideal activity," says Dr. Namey. "It takes the hips, knees, and ankles through a range of motion, without stressing the cartilage." What's more, the gentle range of motion of cycling actually helps to nourish the cartilage, he adds.

Some people with arthritis use an exercise bike to round out their regular fitness program. Lorraine Lamport, for example, rides her stationary bike when bad weather stymies her outdoor walks. And she likes to hop on the bike whenever the osteoarthritis in her knees starts to act up. "It seems like after I ride, my knees improve within a couple of days. I don't know why, but the exercise seems to do something for them. If I'm really stiff and sore, I'll go ride the bike, and the soreness seems to fade," she says.

Researchers report similar effects. At the University of Michigan Medical Center, a group of women with RA pedaled exercise bikes three times a week. No one experienced a joint flare-up or felt worse after cycling. In fact, just the opposite occurred: After 12 weeks, the cyclists had *less* joint pain and swelling. They also had more energy, slept better, and suffered less morning stiffness.

Best of all, because they felt so much better, the women began to do more with their lives. "You would see these people afterward, at the theater, concerts, or a ball game, doing things they'd never done before. Their quality of life was really enhanced," says Richard M. Lampman, Ph.D., one of the scientists who conducted the study.

If you haven't exercised in years, pedaling a stationary bike is a good way to get back in shape, arthritis or no arthritis. An article in the *American Journal of Physical Medicine* tells the story of a middle-aged doctor with RA who pedaled his way back to fitness. He hadn't exercised in 19 years and was worried about his cardiovascular health. After 14 weeks in a cycling program, he lost 7 pounds and lowered his blood levels of cholesterol and triglycerides. His morale also improved because he had accomplished something positive and worthwhile.

Are you wondering if you're a candidate for cycling? If you can stand and walk comfortably, then you can probably cycle, says Dr.

Namey. However, he adds, if you're having a major arthritis flare-up, wait until you feel better before cycling. Also, cycling may be hard—or out of the question—for people with severe arthritis in the lower body. "If you're having extreme pain, don't cycle," he says.

How to Buy and Use a Stationary Bicycle

Before you buy an exercise bike, shop around. Visit a fitness equipment store or two and ask the salespeople to let you test several models. Look for a bike that feels stable and solid as you're pedaling, says Barbara F. Banwell, a physical therapist who was one of the researchers in the University of Michigan cycling study. Also, the bike should have a large flywheel (the front part that spins as you pedal). Some bicycle seats are more comfortable than others, and you may want to exchange an unsatisfactory one for one that's comfortable. Look for a saddle that's wide, cushioned, and adjustable.

The handlebars should be easy to reach from a seated position. If you tend to have back problems, be sure you can sit upright and don't have to bend forward to reach the handlebars. A mechanism to adjust the pedal resistance and gauges for measuring speed, distance, and cadence (revolutions per minute [rpm]) are essential. (If you want to splurge, some models have computer panels on the handlebars that show how many calories you've burned and keep track of your heart rate. But for most people, a less-expensive bike will do.)

If you're using an exercise bike for the first time, here are some guidelines to make your cycling program as safe and effective as possible.

• Adjust the bike to fit you comfortably. Raise or lower the seat so that when each foot is at the bottom of a stroke, the knee of that leg is bent slightly and the foot is at a 90-degree angle to the ankle. Position the handlebars so your arms and shoulders are relaxed.

• Always warm up first by pedaling with no resistance for about 5 minutes.

• After you've warmed up, increase the pedal resistance to a level that seems comfortable but requires some exertion. For your first session, try 5 minutes of cycling with very little resistance. Next time, add a few more minutes of cycling, and increase the resistance slightly so you are pedaling longer and harder each week. Use your target heart rate as a guide to the right level of exertion. Gradually work up to 30 minutes per session three times a week.

● For the last 5 minutes of your workout, cool down by cycling with little or no resistance.

Outdoor Cycling for Fun and Fitness

If indoor cycling starts to become monotonous, take your cycling program outdoors. "You get a chance to look at the countryside," says Dr. Namey, who cycles outdoors on weekends with his wife and two young children. "It takes you off the beaten path. You don't see nearly as much hurtling along in a car going 60 miles an hour as you do from a cycle going 15."

You have plenty of outdoor bikes to choose from. For many people with arthritis, bikes with upright handlebars are more comfortable than those with dropped handlebars, which are designed so that the rider has to lean over. For people with balance problems, an adult tricycle is as much fun but easier to ride than a two-wheeler. And if you have back problems, you might want to consider a recumbent bike, which you ride while reclining, with your feet in front of you.

Just as with a stationary cycle, shop around for an outdoor bike that fits you. Your best approach is to go to several specialty shops that employ knowledgeable salespeople.

When you stand straddling the bike, the crossbar should come almost, but not quite, to your crotch. When you sit in the saddle, your knee should be slightly bent when your foot is extended to the bottom of the pedal stroke. Wider tires will give you a smoother ride, saving your bones from jarring bumps, and upright handlebars will probably be more comfortable than dropped handles if you have arthritis in your hands. (You can also purchase cushioned covers that make the handlebars easier to grip.)

For your first attempt on an outdoor bike, ride on a flat surface in clear, dry weather. A paved path in a park is ideal, since you won't have to worry about automobile traffic. Warm up by walking around for 5 minutes and doing some stretches. Then practice riding in a straight line without swerving, staying in control around curves, and avoiding hazards. For safety, always wear a helmet and use specially designed rearview mirrors, which can be attached to your helmet, glasses, or handlebars.

Occasionally, get off your bike and do a little stretching to keep from getting sore. And periodically check your pulse to see if you're within your target heart rate range, suggests Dr. Namey.

A Troubleshooting Guide to Cycling Pains

If you experience a few mild aches and pains after cycling, don't be alarmed. It's probably not your arthritis flaring up but your body responding to some quirks in your bike. Some minor adjustment may be all that's needed. These suggestions are useful for both indoor and outdoor cycling.

If your knees hurt: Check to make sure the seat is adjusted to the right height. If it's set too high, you could be overextending your legs and straining your knees. Another cause of knee pain is pedaling too hard. If that seems to be the case, pedal faster in a higher gear that requires less force, or slow down. Ideally, you should be in a gear that lets you comfortably pedal at about 70 rpm, says Dr. Namey. To measure your cadence, count how many revolutions you pedal in 15 seconds, then multiply by 4.

If your back hurts: Adjust the seat so you don't have to bend forward to reach the handlebars. If you are riding outdoors, ride on a smooth surface, avoiding bumps and potholes that jar your spine. Also, get off your bike every 15 minutes or so to stretch a bit. Wearing a lumbosacral belt (available at medical supply stores) helps prevent cycling backaches, according to Ronald M. Lawrence, M.D., Ph.D., and Sandra Rosenweig, authors of *Going the Distance.*

If your hands hurt: Ask a bike shop mechanic to adjust the brake levers to make them easier to squeeze. Don't ride with all your weight on the handlebars. Consider wearing padded cycling gloves, and cushion the handlebars by wrapping them with extra padding (available at bike shops). And pull over and stop occasionally to stretch your arms and hands.

If your bottom is sore: Pad the saddle with a Spenco foamlike cover or a sheepskin cover, both available at bike shops. Or you might consider investing in a new saddle. You can choose from anatomical saddles, which conform to your natural shape, sling-type saddles, and even water-filled seats. Check bike shops and the mail-order ads in bike magazines. "You have to experiment to find what's best for you," says Barbara Banwell. "What's right for one person isn't right for another."

Low-Impact Dancing:
No Jumping, Jarring, or Jostling

Do you assume that aerobic dancing is just for people who can take a lot of jumping and bouncing? Not so: People with arthritis can safely work out in modified low-impact aerobic dance classes like everyone else, according to reports.

A group of Chicago researchers, for example, designed an aerobic dance program especially for people with arthritis. "We use a dance format with a traditional warm-up and cool-down," says Susan G. Perlman, M.D., a rheumatologist and assistant professor of clinical medicine at Northwestern University Medical School in Chicago, who directed the study. "The pace is quick, and as a participant myself, I can tell you they get a good workout!"

As in many other low-impact classes, the participants do not run, jump, or bounce. Instead they do slow and fast walking, gliding, swaying, and sliding. In addition, the routine is modified to eliminate stress on wrists or other joints affected by RA. Everyone goes at his own pace and sits in chairs for the warm-up exercises.

Anne Robinson, who has RA and is the associate executive director of the Illinois chapter of the Arthritis Foundation in Chicago, has taken the class on and off for the past six years—and loves every minute of it. "Every time I take that class, I feel sensational," she says. "In fact, you could say I'm hooked on it." When she attends the class regularly, she says, her posture improves, she walks more comfortably, and she has more energy.

Best of all, the classes give Robinson a sense of belonging, a feeling that she can get in shape just like anyone else. "Many times, people with arthritis get bored with the kinds of exercise they've been given," she says. "You want something that's a little more exciting so you can look forward to it and participate in it with others."

In designing the aerobics class, Dr. Perlman and her colleagues wanted to be sure that the vigorous, twice-weekly sessions would not aggravate anyone's arthritis. And it seems to have worked: After 16 weeks, the group felt more energized and in higher spirits. They also could walk faster, and some had less joint swelling and pain. "People did not get worse. On the contrary: In some cases, their arthritis got better," says Dr. Perlman.

Tailoring Low-Impact Dance for Tender Joints

If you can't find a low-impact aerobic dance class for people with arthritis in your community, you may be able to join a general low-impact class if you know your limitations and follow some basic guidelines.

By definition, low-impact classes require that participants keep one foot touching the floor at all times while doing a variety of kicks, side-to-side movements, and lunges. But beware: Just because a class is labeled low-impact doesn't mean it's safe for you. "There are many programs available that are billed as being low-impact aerobics that are *not* low-impact," cautions Dr. Perlman. "And even those that are might not be low-impact enough for arthritic joints."

If you'd like to join a general low-impact aerobics class, here are some guidelines to help you find a safe program and if necessary, modify the routine to make it work for you.

Watch a class once before you sign up. At the first sign of running, jumping, bouncing, or hopping, go elsewhere. Even if the exercises look low-impact, ask the instructor if he can accommodate people with joint problems. Does anyone in the class have knee or back trouble? If so, ask the instructor if you can talk to them to see how they're doing.

Look for a class for mature adults. If some of the participants have a few gray hairs, the class is apt to be more gentle
(continued on page 124)

Finding Fitness Shoes That Fit

Ready to begin a program of walking, low-impact dancing, or other good aerobic exercise? Get off to a good—and safe—start by wearing comfortable, well-cushioned athletic shoes. Footwear made expressly for your chosen activity is ideal.

"If you're going to be exercising, you've got to have good footwear," says Thomas C. Namey, M.D., of the University of Tennessee Medical Center. The right footwear is essential because your shoes serve as shock absorbers, protecting your whole body from injury, not just your feet. Shoes that don't fit, on the other hand, twist your feet out of their natural alignment, throwing off your body mechanics and putting stress on other joints. So the wrong shoes can cause joint problems anywhere from your toes to your shoulders, not to mention abrasions, calluses, and other problems that can get worse with time.

With scores of well-designed fitness shoes on the market, you can find a pair that fits. Here are some general tips on shopping for fitness shoes.

Shop in a good shoe store. Go to a store that stocks a wide selection of athletic footwear and is staffed with well-trained salespeople who really know shoes—and feet—and who will take the time to answer your questions. (Ask coaches, instructors, or exercise veterans where they shop.)

To find shoes that fit well, try, try, try them on again. For the best fit, wear athletic socks to try on shoes. Don't believe any salesperson who tells you that a pair of uncomfortable shoes will feel better after you "break them in." If the shoes fit properly when they're new, they won't bind or chafe.

Take your shoes on a test walk. Don't be fooled by the soft, furry feel of mattress-like insoles as you sit in your chair. The true test of shoes' cushioning ability is how springy they feel when you walk and bounce around in them. Stroll out to the corridor or sidewalk to see how they feel away from carpeted surfaces in the store.

If you wear orthotic devices in your everyday shoes, your fitness shoes should have them as well. Look for shoes roomy enough to fit with the orthotic or shoes with removable insoles. (Naturally, it's best to wear your orthotics when you try on fitness shoes.)

Replace your fitness shoes often.   If you've been exercising for a few months and your knees suddenly start to hurt, you may need a new pair of shoes. Long before your shoes *look* worn out, they may have lost their cushioning quality. To be on the safe side, regular exercisers should replace their shoes every few months.

Here's what to look for when shopping for specialized fitness shoes.

Walking shoes.   Look for a shoe that's lightweight, flexible and well-cushioned, advises Martyn Shorten, Ph.D., director of the Nike Sport Research Laboratory in Beaverton, Oregon. The midsole, which is the shoe's key shock-absorbing component, is sandwiched between the inner sole, which rests against your foot, and the outer sole, which strikes the ground. The midsole alone should be about ½-inch thick in the heel. Also, ask the shoe salesperson what the midsole is made of. The best shock absorbers are polyurethane or EVA (ethylene vinyl acetate copolymer). Midsoles with extra cushioning features, such as pockets of air, are better yet.

Bounce on the heels a few times to make sure the midsoles are springy enough, says Dr. Shorten. Walking shoes should have a roomy toe box, big enough to let you wiggle your toes a bit. Also, look for a flexible shoe that lets your foot roll naturally from heel to toe as you walk.

Aerobic shoes.   Look for a shoe with good cushioning in the forefoot and an outsole that won't slip or drag on gym floors. "If you're walking or running, then most of the impact occurs in the heel," explains Dr. Shorten. "But if you're doing aerobics, then most of the impact goes in the forefoot." If the shoe fits properly, your forefoot will feel stable and not slip from side to side. Look for a smooth rubber outsole, one soft enough for you to make an impression in the material with your thumbnail. A smooth outsole will keep shoes from grabbing a carpeted surface and tripping you or slipping on a wood floor.

Cycling shoes.   Cycling shoes have much stiffer soles than other fitness shoes. They make pedaling more efficient because, when you press down on the pedal, the shoe doesn't bend and no energy is wasted. Cycling shoes generally have less cushioning than other athletic shoes because your feet meet little or no impact. Do choose shoes with adequate heel cushioning, though, so you can walk comfortably when you get off your bike.

than one for younger folks. "If everyone in the class is Miss Body Beautiful or Joe Musclebound, that may not be the class for you," says Dr. Namey.

Check to see whether or not the instructor encourages participants to go at their own pace. That way, if you're having a mild flare-up, you can still participate, as long as you cut back to a less-intense level of exercise.

If a particular exercise bothers you, switch to a safer or easier version of the same activity. If you have trouble lunging from side to side, for example, try stepping to the side instead. If you have RA, avoid exercises that put stress on the small joints of your feet and hands, such as push-ups from the floor, says Dr. Perlman.

When in doubt about an exercise, skip it. Next time you see your physical therapist or doctor, check to see if the exercise is safe for you.

Consider, too, Jazzercise classes, which are mostly low-impact workouts based on jazz dance movements and are recommended by Dr. Namey. Jazzercise classes often work well for people with arthritis because participants go at their own pace and are taught how to modify every exercise with lower-intensity movements. Look in the telephone directory to find a Jazzercise class in your area, write the program's corporate office (Jazzercise, Inc., 2808 Roosevelt Street, Carlsbad, CA 92008), or call 1-800-FIT-ISIT.

Yet another option is no-impact exercise programs, now being run by various hospitals and fitness organizations.

Catch the Wave: Aquatic Exercise

When American astronauts landed on the moon, they bounded along the strange terrain in giant leaps because of the moon's low gravity. You can get a sense of the same low-gravity experience in any swimming pool on earth, where, because of the water's natural buoyancy, your body weighs 90 percent less than it does on land. Thanks to this buoyancy, you can walk—even jog—without painful pounding. And the warmer the water, the better it relaxes and soothes tight, achy muscles and joints.

"The first time I got in the water, I was jumping and dancing because I didn't weigh anything," recalls one woman who regularly attends one of the Arthritis Foundation's aquatic exercise classes. "It was exhilarating. Exercises I can do in water, I can't do on land, because it's too difficult and painful. But I don't have any pain in the water."

And the same water that cushions you also gives you a great workout. Water has greater resistance than air and challenges your muscles to work harder, making them stronger. It's like having a set of weight-training machines right in the pool with you.

And water can buoy your mood as well your body. "I love the water," says Jennifer DePalmer, an accomplished swimmer and pool instructor who has rheumatoid arthritis (RA). "I can be in the crummiest mood and feel physically awful, but if I go and teach a swimming class, I'm fine in an hour. I feel better; my body feels better."

Cushioning, resistance, an emotional lift—and you don't even have to know how to swim. In many aquatic programs, you stand and exercise in the shallow end of the pool, which is usually no deeper than your waist or chest. The pool, of course, is also a natural haven for deep-end exercisers, who can swim laps or play a spirited game of water volleyball.

If you're ready to test the waters, this chapter will show you how to get the most out of pool exercise. Whether you're just getting your sea legs or are an accomplished swimmer, the water offers something for nearly everyone with arthritis.

A Visit to a Water Exercise Class

If you don't like doing range-of-motion exercises on land, take your exercise routine for a dip. In a water exercise class, you do most of the same stretching and strengthening exercises that you would on land. Such classes for people with arthritis are enjoying a tidal wave of popularity. Almost all chapters of the Arthritis Foundation now offer water exercise classes, and some hospitals and fitness centers have started their own programs. "It's very popular," says Michele L. Boutaugh, vice president of patient and community services for the Arthritis Foundation in Atlanta. "We serve more people through our aquatic program than through any another program."

The Mid-City YWCA in Philadelphia has a good example of a class sponsored by the Arthritis Foundation. To most observers, the Y's indoor pool looks clean but ordinary. But to the dozen women with arthritis who come here regularly for the water exercise class, it looks—and feels—like the Fountain of Youth.

As soon as they step into the warm water, their faces brighten with delighted smiles, as though their pains are being washed away. Canes and walkers are left by the side of the pool because in the pool everyone walks more easily. And the rapport among the exercisers is as warm and supportive as the water. "There's a real loving, caring feeling for each other, because we all know what the others are going through," says Sister Marguerite Phillips, a class regular who has osteoarthritis.

For the first 5 or 10 minutes of the class, the women walk back and forth in the shallow end to warm up. Then Wendra Galfand, the class instructor, asks everyone to find a comfortable place to stand. Some hold onto the side of the pool for support, while others stand in water up to their shoulders. Carolyn La Grotta, who is stiff because she hasn't been to class in more than a month, sits on a submerged chair to exercise.

For almost an hour, the water exercisers stretch and strengthen their immersed bodies from shoulders to toes. Some bob and sway to the beat of Barbra Streisand songs in the background. The exercisers become quiet as they intently watch Galfand, but they beam with relaxed smiles. Everyone goes at his own pace, doing only as much exercise as feels right.

When the class ends, no one is in a hurry to leave. Some people stay in the pool to swim laps, others flutter around on kickboards. Back in the locker room, the women talk about how much better they feel because of the pool exercise.

"It's just about the best thing anybody can do for arthritis," says Blanche Weiss, 68, a former dancer. A few years ago, Weiss feared she would be crippled by her severe osteoarthritis and osteoporosis. Now she walks easily and has regained her dancer's grace, thanks to several years of pool work. "It's been a wonderful experience, this water therapy. I don't know what would have happened to me without it. I thought I was going to be an invalid. Now I do just about anything I feel like. I'm going home and putting on my jogging shoes and shorts so I can walk a few miles!"

"The exercise really does wonders," agrees La Grotta. Before she joined the class a year and a half ago, she couldn't stand up long enough to brush her teeth. "Now I can walk about ten blocks. I feel more independent. I feel like a whole person again! I swear by this water exercise. I think I'll come for the rest of my life." (A representative water exercise routine is described in "Water Exercises for Arthritis" on page 128.)

Water Exercises for Arthritis

The water exercises illustrated here are a sampling of what's offered in the Arthritis Foundation YMCA Aquatic Program. If you like these exercises, consider joining a group, where you'll get a more complete workout and have an instructor to guide you.

At first, do only a few repetitions of each exercise and move slowly. As your stamina builds, gradually add more repetitions. On days you don't feel well, cut back to a comfortable level. And remember to warm up first by walking around in the pool for 5 or 10 minutes.

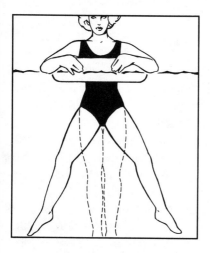

Leg openers. Wear a water ski vest or inner tube around your torso. Point your toes as you spread both legs apart as wide as you comfortably can. Bring them together again. Repeat, with feet flexed.

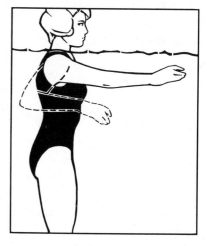

Water rowing. Pretend you're rowing a boat. Extend both arms parallel to the surface of the water. Then bend your elbows, bringing your hands to your chest. Extend your arms again and continue rowing.

Note: These exercises were adapted from the Arthritis Foundation YMCA Aquatic Program, with permission.

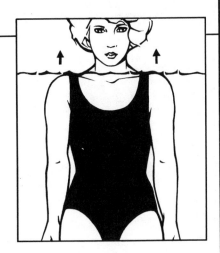

Shoulder shrugs. Stand with the water covering your shoulders, and lift both shoulders up toward your ears. Hold for a few counts. Relax and repeat.

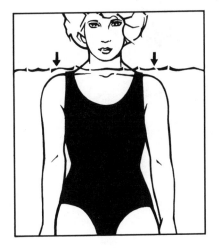

Leg circles. Lift one leg slightly off the pool floor and make small clockwise circles. Then do the same exercise going counterclockwise. Don't cross your leg over the midline of your body. If you need to, hold on to the pool wall for support.

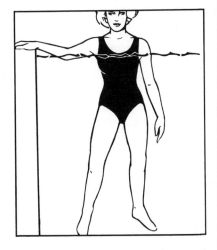

(continued)

129

Water Exercises for Arthritis—*Continued*

Water parade. March around the shallow end of the pool in toy soldier style while swinging your arms without bending your elbows.

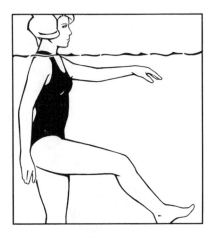

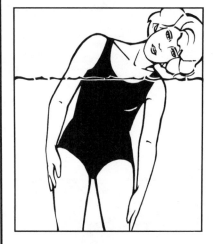

Side benders. Stand in chest-deep water and lean to one side, letting your hand slide down your thigh. Straighten up and repeat on the other side.

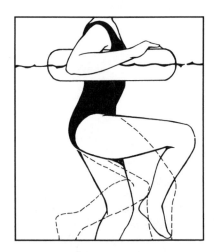

Water cyclist. Wear a water ski vest or inner tube around your torso, and pretend you're on a bicycle. Pedal forward, then backward.

Piano playing. Extend both arms underwater and move them from side to side, imitating a piano player with your fingers as you move.

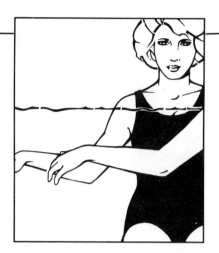

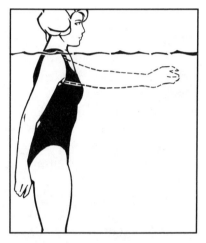

Water applause. Raise both arms to shoulder height and try to clap your hands together. Lower your arms and try to clap your hands behind you.

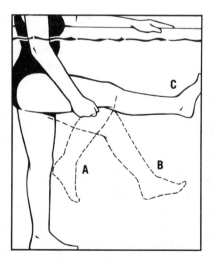

Leg raises. Standing with your back or side against the pool wall, *(A)* bend one knee, keeping your thigh parallel with the surface of the water. Then *(B, C)* straighten the leg. *(A)* Bend the knee again and lower your leg. Repeat with the other leg.

Plunging into Water Exercise

If you're interested in finding a water exercise class, first call your local chapter of the Arthritis Foundation. Most chapters offer a program developed by the national office of the Arthritis Foundation and the YMCA of the USA. A few chapters offer slightly different classes, developed before the national program was introduced in 1983. Classes, which are held in Ys and other community pools, have varying fees, but $2 to $3 per session is typical.

The Arthritis Foundation YMCA Aquatic Program has a lot going for it. Some of the nation's top experts on exercise for arthritis developed the program. Instructors must attend training workshops, where they learn about safe exercise for people with joint problems. And the Arthritis Foundation is picky about which pools offer its classes. The water must be warm—at least 83°F and ideally between 84° and 88°F—and the center must be safe and accessible for people with arthritis. At the Mid-City Y, for example, the pool has a special set of wide steps that make it easy to get in and out.

In some areas, there's a waiting list for the Arthritis Foundation aquatic classes. If you can't attend the foundation's program for some reason, don't get discouraged. Some health clubs, community centers, and even hospitals now offer their own water exercise classes for people with arthritis or back problems. For leads on where to look, check with your local chapter of the Arthritis Foundation, your doctor or physical therapist, and local Ys. (For guidelines on choosing a pool, see "How to Find a Health Club That's Right for You" on page 140.)

If you have a pool at home or prefer to work out alone, you can design your own water exercise routine. But first try to consult with a physical therapist, who can show you the best exercises for your particular condition. (If you don't have a physical therapist, ask your doctor to recommend one who specializes in arthritis.) Until you remember your routine, you might jot down your exercise instructions and enclose them in a plastic binder or Ziploc storage bag that you keep by the side of the pool. (If Ziploc storage bags are a problem for you, you can use a waterproof clipboard.)

Tips for Water Babies

Don't try to make too big a splash your first time in a water exercise class. "People who come in the first time sometimes have a tendency to overdo it, because they feel so wonderful in the water," says Jo Ann Millet, aquatic director for the Central Bucks YMCA in Doylestown, Pennsylvania, and the developer of one of the nation's first water exercise programs for arthritis. "We caution people throughout the whole program: Listen to your body. If it hurts, stop."

If you're afraid of the water, be patient with yourself and look for an understanding instructor who will work with you. That strategy worked for Weiss, who had been terrified of water since the age of three, when her father threw her into a lake in a misguided attempt to teach her to swim. Sixty years later, when her doctor told her she had to try water exercise or face becoming an invalid, she bravely decided to take the plunge. For a long time, she stayed in the shallow end, always keeping her feet firmly on the bottom of the pool and her head well above water. Each time, she'd try to walk in a little bit deeper. With this gradual approach and the gentle encouragement of her instructor, not only did Weiss overcome her phobia, she's also learned to swim. "I'm not afraid," she says. "I love the water exercise now."

When you're getting dressed to go to the pool, think like a quick-change artist. Wear something that's easy to pop on and off, such as a warm-up suit. If you're in a hurry, consider wearing your swimsuit under your clothes. And women should not bother with panty hose, says Millet. "To get a pair of panty hose on a damp body is like doing the Mexican hat dance!" she says. (For more suggestions on pool attire, see "The Well-Prepared 'Pool Shark'" on page 134.)

Aqua-Aerobics Add Challenge

While swimming laps is the first thing that comes to mind for cardiovascular conditioning in the pool, you don't have to know how to swim to get aerobically fit in water. The water's cushioning effect allows some people with arthritis to jog laps, while others attend aqua-aerobics classes in the shallow end.

Whatever activity you choose, warm up first for 5 or 10 minutes by walking around in the pool and doing some range-of-motion exercises for flexibility. Similarly, cool down for the last 5 or 10 minutes by slowing down your pace, then finish with some gentle stretches. If you're out of shape, consult with your doctor about the best aerobic activity for you. Start with as little as 5 minutes of aerobic exercise per session, then gradually increase to 20 to 30 minutes over a period of weeks or months. For maximum

The Well-Prepared "Pool Shark"

Travel light when you're packing up for the pool. Use this checklist to see if you have everything you need.

☐ Swimsuit. Pick a suit that's easy to slip on and off but stays on securely in the water. For women, one-piece suits, especially those with crisscross straps in the back, are best for pool exercise.

☐ Bathing cap. If you don't plan to swim, don't bother with a bathing cap unless the pool requires one. Your hair won't get wet in most Arthritis Foundation water exercise classes—unless someone splashes you. If your hair is longer than shoulder-length, pull it up with a hair band or clips.

☐ Gym bag. Get one that's lightweight and roomy, such as a zippered nylon tote. If you have arthritis in your hands, use a bag with a shoulder strap.

☐ Pool slippers. A pair of sandals or slip-ons with rubber soles will keep you from slipping in a wet pool area or locker room.

☐ Thick terry cloth robe. If the air is drafty around the pool or in the locker room—or if you're too modest to stroll around in just a benefit, try to exercise three times a week. Here are three pool workouts to consider.

Make Waves with Water Jogging

Who says people with arthritis can't run? At the University of Missouri Multipurpose Arthritis Center, researchers found that people with osteoarthritis and RA were able to jog in a pool. The group, which exercised three times a week, ran up some major health benefits: After 12 weeks, they had better cardiovascular fitness, less morning stiffness, and fewer painful, swollen joints.

swimsuit—a robe will keep you from getting chilled.

☐ Towel. If you don't have a robe, a big, bright beach towel will do double duty to cover and dry you. However, if your gym has towel service, don't bother bringing one from home.

☐ Toiletry kit. Buy small sample sizes of your favorite shampoo and lotion just for the gym. Or transfer what you need from big bottles into small plastic ones. Save small bars of free soap from motels for the gym. Keep them all together in a sturdy plastic bag.

☐ Dressing aids. If you need self-help devices to pull on socks, comb your hair, or do other grooming, remember to bring them from home.

☐ Small plastic bag. Keep your wet swimsuit separate from the rest of your gear after your workout by putting it in a plastic bag.

☐ Combination lock. If you use a locker, you need a lock to safeguard your belongings. If you have difficulty manipulating a lock or locker, ask a friend in the class if you can share a space. Some gyms let you bring valuables such as your wallet and car keys out to a visible spot in the pool area for safekeeping.

To get started, try jogging in place in chest-deep water after your warm-up. For more challenging exercise, jog laps from one side of the shallow end to the other. Lap jogging is harder than running in place, because you're pushing your body forward against the water's resistance. Use your target heart rate as a guide to how intensely to exercise. (See chapter 8, "Moving Forward: Aerobic Exercise.") If water jogging is too much exertion for you or causes pain in your legs, try strapping on a water ski vest or other personal flotation device. In the University of Missouri study, some people found that wearing a water ski vest or belt added enough buoyancy to prevent jogging pains. (There is more on flotation devices later in this chapter.) If you can't swim, remember not to venture into deep water, and don't use the pool unless a lifeguard is present.

Water Aerobics Classes

If you really want to kick up your heels in the pool, try a water aerobics, or aqua-aerobics, class. Many health clubs and Ys now offer these challenging water workouts, which are usually geared to people without disabilities. Although these classes are too strenuous for some people with arthritis, others find them a fun and pain-free alternative to aerobic dance classes on land. Jennifer DePalmer, whose RA is in remission, has the energy to teach four water aerobics classes each week in Philadelphia. DePalmer, who can't do aerobic dance on land, can kick and jump with ease in the water. "It's a lower impact," she says. "It provides a lot of support for your joints."

Water aerobics classes vary from pool to pool, but they usually include warm-up, aerobic, and cool-down phases, as well as various exercises for overall toning. Depending on the class, the routine might include water jogging, jumping jacks, can-can kicks, bobbing, treading water, and sometimes a little swimming.

Your arthritis should be well under control before you attempt one of these classes. If in doubt, check with your doctor. Also, you might watch a class before signing up. If it looks safe, try it, but be willing to modify or omit exercises that are too fast, painful, or risky.

Swimming Away from Pain

Swimming, where your whole body rests on a supportive pillow of water, is the ultimate no-impact aerobic exercise. Swimming causes fewer injuries than almost any other recreational exercise, according to a survey conducted by the Gallup Organization. Not surprisingly, swimming has long been touted as *the* aerobic activity for people with arthritis.

But according to people with arthritis who swim, it's truly a case of different strokes for different folks. Depending on what type of arthritis you have, you may need to change your stroke to swim more comfortably and efficiently, perhaps with the advice of a swimming instructor.

"I can't do the Australian crawl like I could when I was a youngster," says Howard J. MacDonald, 68. MacDonald, who has RA, can't do the overhead arm strokes of the crawl because it bothers his shoulders. So, he says, "I do the breaststroke, the sidestroke, and sometimes the dog paddle. You have to keep everything within the range of your body's ability."

The best strokes for people with arthritis are the breaststroke, the sidestroke, and the elementary backstroke, says Louise Priest, executive director of the Council for National Cooperation in Aquatics in Indianapolis. These strokes are easier because they use less range of motion in the upper body than the butterfly or crawl. In the elementary backstroke, for example, the arms stay underwater and never extend above shoulder level. (In the more difficult back crawl, the arms reach all the way out of the water and back over the head.)

If you have neck problems, try the sidestroke or elementary backstroke. Avoid the breaststroke and butterfly, which can hurt your neck, says Valery S. Lanyi, M.D., clinical associate professor of rehabilitation medicine at New York University Medical Center in New York City. If a bad back is the culprit, also try the elementary backstroke, she suggests.

If you want to learn how to swim, or just need some tips on improving your strokes, consider taking lessons with a swimming instructor. "There are very good reasons for working with a swimming instructor," says Priest. "You may be modifying a stroke in such a way as to make it more difficult to do." A swimming instructor can show you how to swim in a style that works best for you.

A Guide to Water Exercise Equipment

To add fun to your water exercise, there's a host of accessories you can take into the pool with you. (Before you invest in these "pool toys," however, check to see what's allowed at your pool.) Here's a guide to what's available at most sporting goods stores.

Kickboards. A kickboard (or swimboard) can help you to cool down after your water workout. Rest your head and hands on the board and lazily flutter-kick your way around the pool. Kickboarding also can be a change of pace from swimming laps.

Mask and snorkel. If arthritis in your neck or back makes it hard for you to turn your head to breathe while swimming, try using a mask and snorkel. You'll be able to breathe without lifting your head out of the water. If you haven't used a mask and snorkel before, ask the pool's water instructor to show you how. It's easy.

Personal flotation vests. A flotation vest (also called a water ski vest or personal flotation device) will buoy you up in either an upright or a swimming position. In the upright position, try "cycling," jogging, or treading water. Sometimes swimmers wear vests for a little added buoyancy or sense of security. Inner tubes and water ski belts, which go around your waist, also add buoyancy.

Hand paddles. These add resistance as you move your arms through the water. Hand paddles make you work harder, but not always better. For some people with arthritis, hand paddles may create too much resistance, putting stress on shoulder and other arm joints. Use them with care, if at all.

Swim fins. Putting fins on your feet can be a fun way to propel yourself through the water. Like hand paddles, however, the wrong fins may create more resistance than you need. Fins that are too long or stiff also can cause muscles to cramp in your legs and feet. Lightweight, flexible fins may be better.

Making a Splash in Your Bathtub

It won't put your neighborhood swimming pool out of business, but a bathtub can become your personal spa for some exercises. Exercising at home in your tub could hardly be more convenient, and you can enjoy water that's much warmer than that in most pools.

What kind of exercises can you do in a bathtub? Everything from neck swivels to torso stretches and toe bends, according to Judy Jetter and Nancy Kadlec, authors of *Bathtub Exercises for Arthritis and Back Pain*. They demonstrate 88 stretching and strengthening exercises to do in a tub, along with a few aerobic exercises such as arm swings and leg cycling.

Some physical therapists are skeptical, however, saying a lot of bathtub exercises are "all wet" in more ways than one. They point out that many people with arthritis have trouble getting in and out of a tub. And unless you plan to turn your bathroom into Sea World, it's almost impossible to submerge your whole body in a tub, so you don't get the water's full benefit. "By the time you get a bathtub deep enough to have the effect of buoyancy, it's probably overflowing," says Kathleen Haralson, a physical therapist and associate director of the Washington University Regional Arthritis Center in St. Louis.

But that doesn't mean all bathtub exercises deserve to go down the drain. The tub is a useful place to do exercises for your submerged hands, feet, and ankles. Depending on how roomy your tub is, you may be able to immerse and exercise other parts of your body as well. If you own or have access to a hot tub or spa, you can do an even wider range of underwater leg and arm exercises. (Check with a reliable financial adviser. The cost of this equipment—or the fee to use it—may qualify as a medical tax deduction.)

Still, most therapists say your bathtub is best used as a relaxing addition to your regular exercise program, not as a substitute for it. Here are three bathtub exercises anyone can try.

Ankle circles. With one leg slightly raised under the water, point your toes and make a circling motion. Then do the other foot.
(continued on page 142)

How to Find a Health Club
That's Right for You

If you plan to join a health club, exercise before you sign up—exercise care, that is. Not all health clubs are suitable for people with arthritis. The poshest club in town won't do you much good if the pool is chilly enough to numb a polar bear or climbing the stairs feels like scaling Pikes Peak.

If you plan to just swim or do water exercises, first check into local YMCAs or Jewish community centers. Memberships are likely to be less expensive than at most private health clubs. Also look into area high schools and colleges, which sometimes open their pools to the public. On the other hand, if you want to pedal an exercise bike one day, swim another, and occasionally do low-impact aerobic dancing, you probably need a full-service health club.

Word of mouth is one of the best ways to find out about suitable fitness centers. If you belong to an arthritis self-help group, ask the group for recommendations about good places to exercise. If you're mainly interested in the pool, ask your local chapter of the Arthritis Foundation where they offer water exercise classes. Even if you just want to swim or exercise on your own, you'll have a list of centers that meet the foundation's standards for safety, accessibility, and warm pool temperature.

Once you have a list of several centers, call them for information and eliminate any that are too expensive, inconveniently located, or lack the particular equipment or programs you're interested in. Then set aside a few hours to visit at least two or three clubs. Here are some questions to ask yourself about each place before you make your final choice.

Is it convenient? The idea is to work up a sweat while you're at the club, not before you get there. Look for a facility near your home or workplace, or perhaps on the route between them. If you can't walk distances, make sure you can park close to the center or use nearby public transportation during the hours you plan to visit.

Is it safe, clean, and accessible? If you don't climb stairs easily, look for a ground-floor center or one with elevators. Check to make sure you can turn shower faucets on and off and open lockers. If you plan to use the pool, see if the steps or ladders are easy to use. Also take a thermometer to check the pool temperature, which can vary throughout the day. (Ideally, the water temperature should be between 83° and 88°F.)

Is the club crowded when you plan to use it?   A pool that is serene and half-empty in midafternoon may be thrashing with lap swimmers or exuberant kids a few hours later. Also, check for lines of people waiting for showers, exercise bikes, or other equipment you plan to use.

What special programs are available?   Even if there are no classes specifically for people with arthritis, you might enjoy a yoga class for relaxation, a ballroom dance class, a low-impact jazz dance class, or swimming lessons.

Are people on the staff well-qualified?   Bulging muscles and sleek thighs don't tell you if an instructor is fit as a teacher. Ideally, aerobics instructors should be certified by one of the several national fitness organizations such as the American College of Sports Medicine or the Institute for Aerobics Research. Pool instructors should be certified by the American Red Cross, the YMCA, or other reputable organization. Find out if any staff members have training in exercise for people with arthritis. Some clubs have a full-time physical therapist on staff, which is a real plus for people who want help designing exercise programs. Staff members should be certified in first aid and cardiopulmonary resuscitation (CPR) methods.

Is the staff interested in you?   Your gut feelings will tell you whether staff members are genuinely enthusiastic about fitness or mostly interested in your checkbook. The better clubs will ask you to fill out a health-risk questionnaire before you start to exercise. Some will evaluate your fitness level and help you to design an exercise program. Instructors should be available to show you how to use equipment correctly or how to modify exercises that are too strenuous.

Do you still like the club after you've tried it once?   Ask for a free pass to the club and try the facility as if you were a regular member. If the club passes this test, you're probably ready to become a full-fledged member. Even so, you may want to opt for a two- or three-month membership before you decide to join for a whole year.

For variety, try drawing numbers from one to ten with your foot pointed in the water.

Cat's claws.   With both hands underwater, slowly bend and straighten your fingers as if imitating a cat's clawing motion.

Toe curls.   With your feet flat against the floor of the tub, curl your toes as if you were picking up a pencil. Hold for a few counts and release.

If you plan to exercise in the tub, keep the water between 85° and 90°F, suggest Jetter and Kadlec. Some people enjoy even warmer water, but don't spend more than a few minutes in a tub hotter than 99°F, because the heat can be stressful for the heart. Note, too, that many hot tubs in health clubs are hotter than 100°F, ruling them out for safe water exercise. (Be careful when emerging from hot water; it dilates the blood vessels in the skin and can make you dizzy unless you climb out slowly.) For bathtub safety, you may want to install tub rails and antiskid strips on the tub floor. Also be sure that no electric appliances, such as hair dryers or radios, are nearby or in a position to fall into the tub.

Using Your Mind
and Emotions to Heal

10

The Three Rs: Relaxation, Rest, and Relief

Marie Stephenson found a way to relieve her arthritis pain that doesn't cost a cent, works in minutes, and is completely safe and natural.

Her "miracle cure"? Relaxation. But true relaxation doesn't mean plopping down on the sofa with a bag of chips to watch soap operas. Whenever her osteoarthritis-ridden back starts to hurt, Stephenson sits down, closes her eyes, and gently coaxes her body into a state of rest—deep, soothing, pain-free rest.

She achieves that rest with a technique called Progressive Relaxation, which involves deliberately tensing and relaxing all her muscles from head to toe. She learned the technique at a clinic by listening to recorded instructions on an audiotape. Invariably, this form of whole-body relaxation helps to relieve her pain. "Relaxation has helped me more than anything I've tried," she says. "It works every time."

There are almost as many ways to relax as there are varieties of arthritis, and you can choose the methods that suit you best. Enjoy the soothing comforts of a warm bath, or use guided imagery to take a mini-vacation from pain without setting foot outside your door. Or, if you're feeling more adventurous, you can try a host of more exotic ways to reduce pain and stress, like spending half an hour in a flotation tank, supported by nothing more than a buoyant cushion of densely salted water.

Whatever methods appeal to you, rest and relaxation are key

components of an arthritis-relief strategy. Stress causes muscle tension that can aggravate arthritis pain, and relaxation is the logical antidote. "If the muscles around a joint are tense, pain and discomfort are amplified," says Mary E. Moore, M.D., Ph.D., director of the Einstein-Moss Rehabilitation Center and professor of medicine at Temple University School of Medicine in Philadelphia. "It becomes a vicious cycle. People feel some discomfort, so they tense up, and the tension causes more pain. Relaxation helps us break that cycle."

Most people with arthritis get the best results by combining two or more pain-control methods, says Susan M. Wright, R.N., D.N.Sc. (doctor of nursing science), a clinical specialist in pain management formerly at Rush Presbyterian/St. Luke's Medical Center in Chicago. For optimal pain relief, she says, it's best to combine medical treatments such as arthritis medications and physical therapy with nondrug pain-management techniques such as those described in this chapter.

Deep-Down-to-Your-Joints Relaxation

"Relax," say your friends. "Go to a movie. Watch a ball game. Do something to take your mind off your pain." But everyday distractions aren't always powerful enough to relax away arthritis pain. For that, you need to reach a deeper level of relaxation, a state of quieted mental activity in which your mind and body are immune to everyday cares.

You've probably experienced such a profound state of relaxation many times without realizing it. Think back to the last time you felt a moment of deep contentment, when your mind was free of troublesome thoughts—riding in a car, perhaps, mesmerized by lovely scenery, or sitting in church, feeling calm and at peace. Imagine how great it would be if you could conjure up deep tranquillity at will.

Well, you can!

The simple techniques that follow enable your mind to switch off the body's customary state of stress. If the techniques are done properly, your heart rate will decrease, you'll breathe more slowly and deeply, and your muscles will relax. And as muscle tension dissolves, you'll find it easier and less painful to move your joints.

Here are a few suggestions to help you get started, no matter what technique you choose.

Find a quiet place to relax that's free of noise and other distractions. Many people with arthritis take frequent rest breaks during the day; these are excellent times to practice a relaxation technique.

Get into a comfortable position. Some people do their relaxation exercises sitting in a chair or recliner, while others lie in bed or sit cross-legged on the floor. Whatever feels good to you is fine. To help you relax, take off your shoes and loosen any tight clothing, like a belt or collar.

Practice. Relaxation is a skill that takes time to learn, like operating a computer or riding a bike. Try to practice twice a day for about 15 to 20 minutes each time, and give yourself at least two weeks to see results.

Progressive Relaxation

Basically, Progressive Relaxation (sometimes called Progressive Muscle Relaxation) involves deliberately tensing, then relaxing, the various muscle groups in your body. The technique was developed years ago by Edmund Jacobson, M.D., who believed that if you wanted to relax, you first had to learn how to recognize when your muscles were tense so you could let go of that tension and relax.

It sounds almost too easy, but Kathleen Kennedy says Progressive Relaxation works wonders for her. Kennedy has osteoarthritis and fibromyalgia, a condition that makes her arms, shoulders, and upper back ache, especially when she's under stress. Before learning Progressive Relaxation, she had no idea that tight, tense muscles aggravated her pain. Progressive Relaxation enabled her to sense when she was becoming tense, so she could relax quickly, before stress-induced pain escalated. "I don't have as many flare-ups now, because I can feel them coming on and I can prevent them by relaxing," she says.

If you'd like to try this technique, here's what to do.

1. Get into a comfortable position, sitting or lying.
2. Close your eyes. Take a deep breath, then exhale very slowly. Repeat.
3. Beginning with your left foot, curl your toes and tighten them, holding for 2 to 5 seconds. Then relax your toes completely, feeling a sense of warmth, tingling, and heaviness. Pay close attention to any differences you feel between when your muscles are tensed and when they are relaxed. Repeat with your right foot.
4. First with your left calf, then with your right, tighten the muscles of each calf for a few seconds, then release the tension. Notice the difference as your legs go limp.
5. Repeat with your left thigh, then your right.
6. Proceed in this way through all the muscle groups in the body. Alternately tighten and relax your buttocks, abdominal muscles, face, neck, shoulders, forearms, hands, and even your forehead.
7. Do a mental check of your body when you've finished the exercise. If any part of your body still feels tense, go back and tense and relax those muscles again.

Caution: If tensing your muscles causes any pain in sore joints, choose another relaxation technique instead. People with rheumatoid arthritis (RA), in particular, may find Progressive Relaxation requires too much energy or causes pain.

Guided Imagery

Guided imagery is like enjoying a mental movie with you as the screenwriter, director, and star. Using the mind's eye as your camera, you can walk along a deserted beach or plunge your hot, achy joints into a cooling mountain stream—without ever leaving home. Focusing on pleasant images helps your body to relax and directs your attention away from pain.

"I've seen some people who have made remarkable changes in how they feel with guided imagery," says Dr. Wright. A favorite image among some of her patients is a vision of themselves sitting in a garden pond, with cool water flowing over their hot joints.

Some forms of guided imagery work as a simple form of relaxation by distracting the mind from pain, giving you a temporary break. Others deal with pain head-on, providing a concrete way to confront—and therefore get rid of—pain by imagining ways to dissolve or diffuse it.

The more powerful the imagery, the greater the potential for pain relief. So be as creative as you like with your mental movies, says Diane Harlowe, occupational therapist and director of occupational therapy and speech services at St. Marys Hospital Medical Center in Madison, Wisconsin, who has taught guided imagery to many arthritis patients. She knows one man who imagines he's packing up his arthritis pain and mailing it away. "In his mind, he actually puts his pain in a box, wraps it up, puts a postage stamp on the box, and mails it to Florida," she says, chuckling. Another man, who works as a trucker, imagines that pain is being pulled out of his back by a Mack truck. And one woman pictures herself riding a rooster while eating a banana—something so absurd it makes the pain more bearable.

To conjure up your own pain-dissolving images:

1. Find a comfortable environment, close your eyes, and focus on your body. Begin to breathe deeply. Let yourself relax.

2. Picture a happy occasion in your life, perhaps a visit to a favorite vacation spot, a ride on a porch swing from your childhood, walking on a serene beach at sunset, or a stop at a secluded waterfall. Pay close attention to your imaginary surroundings: Details make imagery more powerful. If you are outside, note the season and the weather. What's the temperature? Is it warm or cool? Is it damp or dry? Look all around you: Are other people nearby? Pay attention to sounds, smells—and taste. If something to eat or drink is part of the image, savor the taste and texture in your mouth. Enjoy your surroundings. When you're ready, slowly bring your thoughts and feelings back to the room you're in. You will feel calm and refreshed from your imaginary journey and ready to open your eyes.

Deep Breathing Exercises

You can't find a much easier way to relax than stopping to take a few deep breaths. Slow, deep breathing is the way nature intended us to breathe. With deep breathing you use your diaphragm and abdominal muscles to expand your lungs more fully, helping to calm nerves and supply the body with oxygen. In contrast, people who take short, shallow breaths, moving air in and out of just the top quarter of their lungs, may not get enough oxygen and may feel fatigued as a result.

Here's how to breathe deeply: Sit up straight, resting your hands lightly on your abdomen. Now slowly inhale through your nose. As you breathe in, you should feel your abdomen begin to expand like a balloon. Next, slowly exhale through your mouth, feeling your abdomen contract.

As you exhale, imagine yourself blowing at a candle strongly enough to cause flickering but not strongly enough to blow it out.

To achieve relaxation, it's important to focus attention on your breathing, concentrating deeply on the in/out flow. Repeat this slow and easy deep breathing exercise a few times, then sit quietly for several minutes as you breathe normally again. (Once you get the hang of it, you might practice abdominal breathing throughout the day, which will help give you more energy and reduce stress. The idea is to adopt abdominal breathing as your regular breathing pattern, so that you automatically breathe this way.)

If you'd like to learn self-help relaxation exercises like these in a group setting, call your local chapter of the Arthritis Foundation and ask if any programs are available in your area. Many chapters teach relaxation exercises as part of a regular arthritis self-help course, which also teaches a variety of coping skills. Or you can also purchase audiotapes with complete instructions for guided imagery, Progressive Relaxation, and other relaxation techniques from the Stanford Arthritis Center. For costs and other ordering information, write to Stanford Arthritis Center, HRP Building, Room 6, Stanford, CA 94305.

Learning to Relax with Beeps, Batteries, and Buoyancy

Some relaxation techniques are a little more elaborate, require special equipment, or require instruction from psychologists or other qualified professionals. While you may need supervision to learn them initially, the benefits can carry over to everyday life for months afterward.

Biofeedback

If you have trouble learning relaxation methods, ask your doctor, a nurse, or a physical therapist about biofeedback. Biofeedback is simply learning how to relax while hooked up to a sensitive monitoring device. The equipment, which can measure your heart rate, skin temperature, or other body changes, helps you to distinguish whether your muscles are tight or relaxed. Marie Stephenson, for example, learned her relaxation exercise while hooked up to a biofeedback machine. Whenever she became tense, the machine detected a change in her skin temperature and beeped steadily. This information helped her realize she was tensing up. As soon as she relaxed, the machine stopped beeping.

After five or six sessions at the clinic, Stephenson found she was able to relax on her own, without being hooked up to the machines. Now she can relax at home automatically, simply by sitting in a chair and focusing her attention on subtle body changes. She no longer needs feedback to remind her how to relax. (Other people may need to continue to listen to an audiotape with a relaxation exercise to help them to remember how to relax at home.)

There are many versions of biofeedback, but all work essentially by showing you how your body reacts to stress and how to control your body responses.

TENS

In ancient Rome, one well-meaning physician treated gout by attaching electric eels to his patients' painful joints. For some, the resulting jolt provided temporary pain relief. But others suffered a very serious side effect: fatal electric shock.

Sound fishy? Maybe so. But physicians are again using electricity to treat arthritis pain. This time, however, the method is safe, sophisticated, and effective. It's called TENS, for transcutaneous (across the skin) electrical nerve stimulation. TENS transmits brief pulses of electricity through the skin to the nerve endings that carry pain messages to the central nervous system.

Two theories explain how TENS works. The device may block the transmission of pain impulses from the tissues to the central nervous system. Or TENS may control pain by stimulating the production of endorphins, morphinelike substances that are made by nerve cells and block pain signals. Some say TENS works both ways.

However it works, TENS is convenient. You can wear the battery-operated device—which is about the size of a garage door opener or beeper—at home, work, or play. Wires from the device lead to small electrodes, which are adhesive-backed or are attached to the skin with adhesive tape at the sites of pain. The TENS unit can be attached to your belt or tucked in a pocket, and the wires are hidden under clothing. Most people turn the machine on and off according to guidelines recommended by a doctor or physical therapist. You can adjust the machine to provide just the right voltage and frequency of pulsation for your needs.

TENS can be used for almost every type of arthritis, says Theresa M. Meyer, R.N., a TENS therapist in Minneapolis who trains both patients and other health care professionals to use the device. "The typical TENS user with arthritis has osteoarthritis in the lower back or knees, but it can be used in any joint," she says. The degree of pain relief varies from person to person. Some people feel better as soon as the device is turned on, while others must use TENS for several days or weeks before experiencing maximum relief. However, about a third of arthritis patients who try TENS don't find it useful for pain relief, she adds. In those for whom TENS does work, it's used in tandem with other pain-management techniques.

JoAnne Haning uses TENS to help relieve arthritis pain in her lower back, which sometimes is so severe she has to stay in bed. On some days, she says, turning on the TENS unit makes her feel well enough to get up and fix her own lunch. But on other days, not even TENS can relieve her terrible pain. "I've been pleased with TENS, but it hasn't been 100 percent effective in relieving my pain," she says.

In any event, TENS doesn't cause additional pain or discomfort if used properly, Meyer says. Haning says she feels a pleasant tingling when the machine is on. Other patients describe an acceptable tapping or massaging sensation.

Although TENS has some impressive potential benefits, it has a few limitations. Some people develop rashes near where the electrodes touch the skin, although the problem usually clears up when the electrodes are repositioned or changed. TENS also cannot be used by people with cardiac pacemakers, because the electrical impulses from the TENS unit may interfere with the pacemaker's signals. In fact, anyone with an unstable heart problem should use TENS cautiously, and pregnant women should not use TENS at all.

TENS users also should take care not to get their units soaking wet, because water can damage the device. But users need not worry about being electrocuted if they get caught in a sudden rain shower or splashed at a backyard pool. At worst, the user will feel an unpleasant—but harmless—tingling, due to water conducting electricity around the skin. Turning the device off will stop the sensation.

If you'd like to try TENS, talk to your doctor, nurse, or physical therapist. If TENS is suitable for your pain problem, a therapist will show you exactly how to use the machine. Most people rent a TENS unit on a trial basis for a month, then decide whether to continue using the device. (You can either continue to rent or buy your own unit.) If you decide to rent or buy a unit, check your medical insurance policy, which may cover all or part of the cost. (A good-quality unit costs about $600.)

Flotation Tanks

Want to really get away from it all? Try floating for an hour in a float tank. From the outside, a float tank looks like a giant egg. Inside, you lie on a shallow pool of densely salted water, so buoyant that you float like a cork. After an hour in this soothing, weightless environment, the typical floater feels about as much anxiety as a damp dishrag.

Sound like it's only for sci-fi fans? Hardly. A number of scientific studies have shown that regular sessions in a flotation tank (flotation therapy) can produce profound relaxation. What's more, flotation therapy (also called Restricted Environmental Stimulation Therapy, or REST) can provide excellent pain relief for some people with arthritis.

So say two researchers at the State University of New York at Stony Brook, who found that a group of RA patients felt significantly less pain after floating. The 15 patients floated for an hour twice a week for six weeks. "The majority of patients felt pain relief as soon as they got out of the tank," says researcher Craig Lehmann, a clinical chemist and associate professor in the school's Department of Medical Technology. Many patients said that once they became accustomed to the therapy, their pain relief continued for three or four days after each treatment.

Clifton Mereday, the physical therapist who collaborated on the study, says that many patients also became more mobile and active after floating, probably because of their lessened joint pain. He recalls an 83-year-old woman in particular, who came to her first float in a wheelchair: "She was really depressed when she first came in. She said she didn't feel like living anymore, the way she hurt." To the researchers' astonishment, after a few sessions in the float tank, the woman walked in one day (no wheelchair!) smiling and wearing lipstick. "Not only was she able to walk, but her depression had lifted because she felt more self-reliant," says Mereday. "She started lecturing everyone about how important it was not to give up!"

One floater describes the sensation as being like floating in space. You can float in the dark, or if you prefer, turn on a light inside the tank or prop the tank door open. And many tanks come with a speaker system to pipe in your favorite relaxing music.

Mereday believes that flotation reduces RA pain by relieving stress, thus relaxing tight muscles and easing joint pain. In addition, Lehmann speculates that soaking in the tank's saturated solution of Epsom salts may directly reduce joint swelling by drawing water out of the body. (A rheumatologist we consulted, however, says there's no evidence to support that theory.)

However it works, you're free to try float therapy yourself—if you can afford it. Many communities now have commercial flotation centers, where you can float for $20 to $35 an hour. Usually, you get a private room with a float tank and a shower. The water inside the tank is heated to body temperature, so you feel neither warm nor cold. The recommended way to float is in the nude, but of course you're free to wear a swimsuit if you wish.

If you can't locate a flotation center in your area, write to Enrichment Enterprises, Inc., 77 Cedar Street, Babylon, NY 11702. Or call the company at 1-800-FLOAT-88. The company, a leading manufacturer of float tanks, keeps an updated list of float centers nationwide and is glad to answer questions about floating.

Acupuncture: Mixed Results from an Ancient Healing Art

What would you say if your doctor stuck a needle in your ear to relieve a pain in your knee? Well, you might say thank you, because it just might work. Physicians who practice the ancient Chinese healing art of acupuncture believe that inserting hair-thin needles at precise locations on the skin can treat everything from arthritis pain to stomach gas, even though the needles may be far away from the site of pain.

According to Chinese philosophy, acupuncture works by restoring the balance of energy in the body. This energy or life force, called Ch'i (pronounced "key"), moves through the body along specific pathways called meridians. Ch'i must flow freely for good health. If the energy flow becomes blocked or impaired because of stress or other factors, pain and illness may result. Acupuncture works, it's said, by stimulating specific points on the meridians, thus helping to restore the flow of energy and alleviate pain.

Typically, the acupuncturist inserts the sterilized, stainless steel needles into the skin for about 20 to 30 minutes. As incredible as it may sound, most people say they feel no pain from the needles, just a faint tingling or heavy sensation. The needles, which have rounded edges, are usually eased into the skin without drawing blood.

Western doctors view acupuncture differently. They say acupuncture works much like TENS, by stimulating the production of endorphins and interfering with the transmission of pain messages from the tissues to the central nervous system.

David E. Bresler, Ph.D., executive director of the Bresler Center in Santa Monica, California, and author of *Free Yourself from Pain,* tells the story of watching a master acupuncturist treat a man in his late 60s who had severe osteoarthritis in his hands. The man's knuckles were swollen to the size of walnuts, and he was in such pain that it was difficult even to examine him. The acupuncturist put needles in the man's hands, as well as his back, ears, and feet. "About 2 minutes after the last needle was inserted, the man began to move his fingers slowly," Dr. Bresler reports. "His eyes opened wide as he exclaimed, 'My God, the pain is gone! It's a miracle!' "

As compelling as this story may be, scientific studies on the use of acupuncture for arthritis show mixed results. In one study, people with RA got some pain relief from acupuncture, but the treatment didn't help their joint swelling or range of motion. Still other studies have failed to confirm the reported benefits of acupuncture for chronic low back pain, tendinitis, and bursitis.

Moreover, acupuncture can be risky if performed by an incompetent acupuncturist, warns Dr. Mary Moore of Einstein-Moss Rehabilitation Center. If the needles are not carefully sterilized after use, they can spread infection among patients. If, for example, the acupuncturist accidentally punctures a patient's skin with a contaminated needle, germs on the needle may enter the person's blood. Conceivably, says Dr. Moore, those germs could transmit AIDS or hepatitis.

Dr. Moore, who has done research on acupuncture, prefers TENS to acupuncture. TENS is safer and can be used at home, while acupuncture requires repeated trips to an acupuncturist, she says. "Most medical doctors would probably say that acupuncture is a very crude, very antiquated, and very inefficient way of providing anybody with pain relief."

Nonetheless, some people with arthritis do get some pain relief from this treatment, says Dr. Wright. If you want to try acupuncture, make sure you choose a qualified practitioner, ideally a physician with experience in treating your type of problem. One source for names of certified licensed practitioners is the National Commission for the Certification of Acupuncturists. This group certifies practitioners who pass an examination and, according to the commission's standards, are qualified to practice acupuncture. For a small fee, the organization will send you a list of acupuncturists in your general area. For details, write to them at 1424 16th Street NW, Suite 105, Washington, DC 20036.

The Therapeutic Power of Touch

It feels so good when someone gives you a hug, a back rub, or just a consoling touch on the arm. Well, there's more to those good feelings than meets the eye. The healing power of human touch is the basis for an unconventional pain-management technique called therapeutic touch, which is practiced mainly by nurses.

Therapeutic touch is based on the idea that each of us is surrounded by an invisible energy field, which extends beyond the level of the skin. "We've all experienced this energy field without realizing it," says Dr. Wright, who has done clinical studies on therapeutic touch and used the method on arthritis patients. "Perhaps one of the most familiar examples is the feeling of having your 'space invaded' while standing with others in a crowded elevator, even though you might not be making physical contact with anyone."

Dr. Wright says that pain from arthritis and other illnesses can disturb this energy field and that by restoring the energy field to normal, the practitioner can help relieve the pain. The first step, though, is to assess the person's energy field. The nurse holds her hands a few inches above the person's head and moves them down each side of the body. With her hands, she tries to detect sensations, such as heat or tingling, that may signal a disturbance in the field and corresponding pain. If trouble spots are detected, the nurse tries to treat the problem by moving her hands in a way that "smooths out" the energy field. The nurse may or may not touch the person's body directly during the procedure. In fact, many practitioners purposely avoid touching the skin because it interferes with their ability to sense the energy field, says Dr. Wright.

And therapeutic touch does help to relieve pain in some arthritis patients, according to Dr. Wright. "It works better for some conditions than for others, and it tends to work extremely well for acute flare-ups of RA," she says.

Whether or not an "energy field" is involved, therapeutic touch can produce deep muscle relaxation, says Dr. Wright. "If someone has chronic pain that's not relieved by therapeutic touch, you can at least make them more relaxed so they feel better." (One rheumatologist we consulted said, "It certainly sounds safe, as long as it's combined with traditional medications.")

Nationwide, close to 7,000 nurses practice therapeutic touch, usually in conjunction with other pain-management methods. To find a nurse or other health professional in your area who's skilled in this healing art, write to Nurse Healers Professional Associates, 175 Fifth Avenue, Suite 3399, New York, NY 10010.

Hot and Cold Tips for Pain Control

A change in the temperature of an affected joint can also relieve pain. Surprisingly, applying either heat or cold may soothe your discomfort, depending on what you prefer and what type of arthritis you have. Even on sweltering summer days, for example, Kathleen Kennedy swaddles her aching arms in warm compresses. Gwen Ellert, on the other hand, says there's nothing like a bag of frozen peas—applied, not eaten—to comfort a hot, painful joint. Yet others have it both ways: They get the best relief from arthritis pain by alternately plunging their sore joints into warm, then cold, water.

So what should it be: Heat? Cold? Both? How can opposites like heat and cold *both* work for arthritis pain? The answer is, it depends. Here are some guidelines for deciding which is better.

Hot Joints? Go for the Cold

"If a joint is hot, swollen, and painful, you don't want to do anything that's going to increase the temperature of that joint. You want to draw the heat out of the joint," says Victoria Gall, a physical therapist and clinical specialist in rheumatology at Brigham and Women's Hospital in Boston. Cold temporarily numbs pain and reduces swelling.

So if you're having a flare-up of RA, you're better off applying cold treatments to painful, swollen joints, she says. (Cold is usually recommended to ease pain and swelling after minor joint injuries, such as a twisted ankle.)

A Few Words of Caution
about Heat and Cold

When used properly, heat and cold are safe for most people with arthritis. But as with any medical treatment, you should observe some safety tips.

- Don't apply heat or cold for extended periods. Most physical therapists say 20 minutes at a time is the safe limit for either treatment.
- With either cold or hot packs, wrap the pack in a light towel (or pillowcase) to protect skin and other tissues from damage.
- If you use heat, test the temperature first; the heat treatment should feel comfortably warm, but not burning hot.
- Don't use an arthritis cream with a heating pad. Mentholated, methyl salicylate arthritis and muscle-ache creams like Ben-Gay carry label warnings against their use in combination with a heating pad.

One California man found out the hard way why the last warning should be heeded.

According to his doctor, the man had applied the cream to his arms and legs, then used a heating pad for several minutes at a time for a total

---

Doctors and therapists often recommend the following cold treatments to relieve arthritis pain. (Before you try either cold or heat treatments, though, you should read "A Few Words of Caution about Heat and Cold" above.)

Homemade ice packs. A bag of frozen vegetables makes a handy cold pack. When you're done, toss the bag of vegetables back into the freezer to reuse another day. (Just don't eat them.) Or make your own cold pack by putting ice cubes inside a Ziploc storage bag, and then putting the sealed bag inside another Ziploc storage bag for extra protection from leakage. A hot- water bottle also can be filled with crushed ice and water. Apply cold treatments for 10 to 20 minutes at a time.

of 15 to 20 minutes of heat at each site. (He claimed not to have fallen asleep using the pad.)

The next day, the man developed large blisters on his arms and legs. Three days later, when the dead skin was removed, doctors discovered that his skin had been destroyed all the way down to the muscles. The man required skin grafts and spent nearly a year in the hospital. He sustained permanent damage to his skin and kidneys.

"Heat makes skin absorb so much of the cream that it becomes toxic," says Madeline C. Y. Heng, M.D., of the Veterans Administration Medical Center, Sepulveda, California. "People need to know just how serious this injury can be."

Finally, a few people may not be able to use heat or cold treatments at all. Check with your doctor if you have impaired temperature sensation, fragile skin, or circulatory problems caused by diabetes or other illnesses. Arthritis sufferers who also have Raynaud's phenomenon, a disorder in which the fingers turn blue and white after exposure to cold, must also avoid cold treatments.

Cold water soaks. Soaking hands or feet in a bucket or sink of cold water (about 65°F) for 15 to 20 minutes may also help.

Reusable cold packs. Chemical cold packs, used as first aid by some hospital emergency rooms, are sold in pharmacies and medical supply stores. Gel-filled packs, which mold around a sore area, are most convenient, although they're more expensive than homemade cold packs. They can be frozen for later reuse.

Some Like It Hot

Unless their joints are already hot and painful, most people with arthritis prefer heat, says Gall. And no wonder. Heat treatments are good for body and soul. If you have morning stiffness, for example, a warm shower or bath helps to loosen up the connective tissues around joints, making you more limber. Heat also can temporarily relieve pain by relaxing tense muscles, thus easing pressure on joints. And nothing beats the soothing tranquility of a warm bath to relax jangled nerves.

Physical therapists say that heat treatments can be applied to any sore joint or muscle, as long as tissues aren't actively inflamed (that is, hot, swollen, and red). Here are some heat treatments they recommend.

Electric heating pad. Make sure any pad you use has a temperature control dial, not just an on/off button, to prevent overheating. Never use a heating pad on the highest setting. To further prevent burns, do not lie on top of or fall asleep on a pad that's plugged in. (Always read the instructions for safe use that accompany a heating pad.) If you prefer moist heat, look for a heating pad specially designed to accommodate a moistened piece of terry cloth. (Such pads are available in major retail stores).

Hot-water bottle. Don't overlook the time-honored hot-water bottle. (Be sure to follow the directions to the letter.)

Hydrocollator pack. This is a canvas bag containing silicone gel, which gives off heat longer than warm compresses. To use a hydrocollator pack, you first heat the silicone containers in boiling water, then wrap the pack in six to eight layers of towel (to protect your skin from burns) and apply it to a painful joint. Like hot-water bottles, hydrocollator packs are available in pharmacies and medical supply stores.

Long bath or soak in a Jacuzzi. You can relax tight, sore muscles and joints in water that's comfortably warm (but not above 100°F, especially if you have high blood pressure or a heart condition). If you have trouble getting into and out of the tub, install tub rails, available in medical supply stores. And everyone—not just arthritis sufferers—should line the bottom of his tub with nonskid strips or a rubber mat, says Gall. (If you can manage it safely, a soak in a Jacuzzi or other kind of hot tub might feel good, too.)

Warm shower. Many arthritis sufferers enjoy using a hand-held shower with a massage unit and directing the stream on their sore joints. If you have trouble standing, install a shower bench so you can sit.

Hot-and-Cold Relief

Some people find that the contrast of alternating between warm and cold treatments is most effective in relieving arthritis pain. To take a contrast bath, fill one container with warm water and another with cool water. Put your hands or feet in the warm water for 3 minutes, then switch to the cool water for 1 minute. Repeat this procedure two or three times, ending with warm water.

Better Sleep, Less Pain

Are you wide awake at 3:00 A.M., counting your aching joints instead of sheep? Do you awaken before dawn, long before you plan to arise? Do you toss and turn so much at night that you feel like a human wave machine?

If so, you have plenty of bleary-eyed company. "We've found that people with arthritis have more sleeping difficulties (delays in falling asleep or awakening in the middle of the night) than people without arthritis—even if the people without arthritis suffer problems such as low back pain," says Stephen Wegener, Ph.D., a clinical psychologist and sleep researcher who works with arthritis patients at the University of Virginia Health Sciences Center in Charlottesville. "We've also found that an arthritis sufferer who has difficulty sleeping will have more severe pain during the day." Sleep problems and pain are intertwined in a vicious cycle, he adds. "People who have the worst sleep have the worst arthritis pain. And people who have the worst pain have the worst sleep."

If you suspect your sleep habits are below par, ask yourself the following questions.

• Does it usually take me more than half an hour to fall asleep at night?

• Do I habitually wake up more than four times at night?

• Do I frequently wake up in the early morning hours, before my customary rising time, and have trouble going back to sleep?

If you answer yes to any of those questions, and you have arthritis, your sleep habits and your arthritis may be affecting each other.

In one study, Dr. Wegener and his colleagues showed that people with various kinds of arthritis woke up an average of six times during the night, twice as often as other people of the same age and sex who didn't have arthritis. Those findings don't surprise Dorothy Withrow, who says her RA frequently keeps her awake at night. "I used to be a very good sleeper. I would reach up to put the light out, and before my head was back down on the pillow I'd be asleep—and I'd sleep through the night," she says. "Now I often awaken two, three, or four times a night."

What causes these unsolicited wake-up calls? "Pain and depression are the chief culprits," says Dr. Wegener. Although people who wake up in the middle of the night usually think they just need to go to the bathroom, it's often pain that awakens them in the first place, he says. Depression, too, can often disturb sleep, typically by waking a person up around dawn. Pain- and depression-triggered sleep disturbances are compounded by advancing age: As we age, we tend to sleep less and wake up more often.

"Unfortunately," says Dr. Wegener, "if you develop poor sleep habits, it may prolong the length of an arthritis flare-up or keep you from recovering from arthritic episodes as quickly." Without restful sleep, it's harder to cope with arthritis during the day, he adds. And people who are constantly awakened during stages of deep sleep may develop symptoms of fibromyalgia, a syndrome that causes muscles and joints to feel achy and stiff, compounding the discomfort of their arthritis.

How can you tell if your sleep habits are affecting your arthritis? "Ask yourself how you feel during the day," advises Albert Wagman, M.D., chief of neurology and associate director of the Sleep Disorders Center at Abington Memorial Hospital in Abington, Pennsylvania. "If you feel rested and alert throughout the day, then you shouldn't worry about your sleep," he says. "On the other hand, if you have trouble staying awake during the day, then you're in trouble."

Nine Tips for Sounder Sleep

If you feel trapped in the pain/insomnia cycle, take heart. The answer may be surprisingly simple. One of Dr. Wegener's patients, for example, suffered from insomnia partly because she drank half a dozen cans of caffeine-containing colas in the evening. By cutting out the cola and learning more healthful sleep habits, she shortened the time it took her to fall asleep from 90 minutes to less than 10 minutes. And she no longer experienced early-morning awakenings. Best of all, she felt more rested and cheerful during the day and had less arthritis pain.

The following tips for getting a good night's sleep come from Dr. Wegener and other sleep experts. If these strategies don't seem to help, talk to your doctor—he will let you know if you have a sleep disorder that can be treated medically. If depression disrupts your sleep, for example, antidepressant medications or therapy may help to restore your sleep (and your spirits).

Go to bed and get up at the same time each day, even on weekends and holidays. Maintaining a regular schedule keeps your natural sleep rhythms in sync, so you'll naturally feel drowsy at bedtime and alert when you wake up.

Don't eat, read, or watch television in bed. "We tell people with sleep problems that they shouldn't do anything in bed but sleep and have sex," says Dr. Wegener. "The idea is that people who have sleep problems no longer associate their bed with sleep the way they should." In other words, if you habitually use your bed for activities like reading or eating snacks, just lying motionless in bed no longer promotes sleep.

If you can't fall asleep within 20 minutes, don't force it. Instead, get up and do something else, like watching a boring television show or reading something dull. As soon as you start to feel sleepy, go back to bed. If you still can't fall asleep, get up after another 20 minutes and repeat the procedure. It sounds like a lot of bother, says Dr. Wegener, but this trick actually works quite well to break the worry/insomnia cycle. If you lie in bed only when you're sleepy, you won't associate your bed with worry and insomnia. (Try this diversionary tactic if you wake up in the middle of the night and can't get back to sleep, too, suggests Dr. Wegener.)

If you feel arthritis pain before bedtime, do something to take the edge off. Soak in a warm bath to soothe muscle tension, or ask a family member for a gentle massage. If you take arthritis medications, ask your pharmacist or physician if you can time one of your regular doses for bedtime to ease any pain that might keep you awake.

Learn deep breathing or other relaxation exercises to keep stress from robbing you of sleep. Many of Dr. Wegener's patients practice relaxation exercises three times a day: morning, afternoon, and before bed. If you wake up at night and can't fall asleep, try a relaxation technique again, he suggests.

Make your bedroom as conducive to sleep as possible. To stay warm, some folks with arthritis get inside a sleeping bag placed under a blanket. Electric blankets are also warming, especially if you preheat them for 10 or 15 minutes before bedtime. Select a mattress that's comfortable for you; some people like a firm mattress, while others go for a water bed. Try to eliminate any noise or lights that might disturb your sleep. (On the other hand, some people sleep better with neutral background noise, like the hum of a fan.)

If you have trouble falling asleep, don't take naps during the day. Daytime naps can interfere with the quality of your sleep at night. Instead, take a relaxation break. Or perk up your spirits with a walk, a swim, or bicycling. People who exercise regularly usually sleep better and are bothered less by pain. (Avoid any type of vigorous exercise for several hours before bedtime, though. It may leave you too revved up to sleep.)

Avoid caffeine, alcohol, or heavy meals before bedtime. The caffeine in coffee, tea, cocoa, and cola drinks can keep you awake, so it's best to avoid these products after 6:00 P.M. And while a glass of wine or beer may make you feel drowsy at first, alcohol's aftereffects can awaken you later at night. So avoid alcoholic beverages for several hours before bedtime. If you're hungry before bed, a light snack is fine, but a heavy meal may interfere with sleep.

In general, avoid over-the-counter sleeping pills. Sleeping pills lose their effectiveness within two or three weeks and can be habit-forming (that is, you can no longer get to sleep without them), says Dr. Wagman. If you feel you need medication to help you sleep, talk to your doctor. (Sleeping pills are for *occasional* relief—they're not a solution to insomnia.)

11

Positive Healing:
Using Your Emotions
to Control Pain

Kathleen Lewis isn't psychic, yet she can often predict when her arthritis will flare up. During her long and emotionally wrenching divorce, for example, she discovered that whenever she got angry or upset and tried to suppress her feelings, she'd soon have problems. "I would have a flare-up within two or three days."

Lewis has more than one form of arthritis. But as a registered nurse and psychotherapist, she knows a thing or two about managing her emotions. Now, whenever she gets really upset, she lets herself have a good cry to vent her feelings of frustration. "I find that if I just let it all out, if I cry, moan, groan—and beat a pillow if need be—I can head off a flare-up."

For better or for worse, says Lewis, her emotions affect her health to a remarkable degree. And doctors say she isn't unusual. For one thing, arthritis can be aggravated by stress, whether it's a major event such as losing your job or a rash of everyday hassles such as sitting in a traffic jam and being late for work. Anxiety, fatigue, fear, and depression—along with a host of other negative emotions—can make your arthritis feel worse and rob you of a full and happy life.

Scientists have just begun to explore the connections between arthritis and emotions. They know that, in general, emotions can change body chemistry and have other physical effects. Stress, for example, can cause pain by making muscles tight and tense. Emotions also influence how your mind perceives pain. If you worry or feel depressed, you may focus your attention on your pain, which makes you feel even worse. On the other hand, if you feel confident and optimistic, you may be better able to control pain.

You don't have to look far to find the one person who can best help lift your spirits. It's *you*. "The first step toward emotional and spiritual health is assuming responsibility for yourself," says Lewis, who's written a book called *Successful Living with Chronic Illness* and now counsels others with arthritis. "You can choose what you're going to focus on in any given situation, including your fight against arthritis. You can choose to be angry or hurt or depressed—or you can choose not to be."

This chapter will show you how to become more adept at managing your emotions. By learning how to cope with stress and eliminate depression and fatigue, you can begin to put more positive emotions to work for you.

A "Can-Do" Attitude Works Wonders

If feeling down in the dumps makes arthritis feel worse, can a spunky attitude have the opposite effect? A number of psychologists say yes. Several studies have shown that people with arthritis who adopt a "can-do" attitude, a sense of confidence in their ability to manage their arthritis, actually suffer less pain and disability. "People who have that can-do attitude are more likely to get out of their chairs and do things, like living more independently and participating more fully in life," says Christopher Lorish, Ph.D., assistant professor of education and medicine at the University of Alabama School of Medicine, Birmingham.

How can you feel "up" in the face of a downer like arthritis? For starters, you can take up a challenging pursuit that will make you feel more confident and successful. That's the secret of a remarkable program offered at Northwestern University in Chicago, where people with rheumatoid arthritis (RA) are proving that they can do whatever they set out to do. They start out with a low-impact aerobic dance class called Educize. Vigorous exercise not only keeps the participants fit, it also gives them confidence in their ability to accomplish what most others with RA would assume is impossible.

After the twice-weekly exercise classes, the participants meet for an hour to brainstorm how they can apply their growing self-confidence to new pursuits. "We encourage people to dream about goals they thought were impossible to achieve because of their arthritis," says Karen Connell, a Chicago educational consultant who, with Susan Perlman, M.D., a Northwestern rheumatologist, helped develop the program. "They begin to very actively develop and explore their fantasies. And they create ways for themselves to be able to do that."

One participant, Barbara, was very disabled by serious RA and could no longer work. Her dream was to travel by train from her home in Chicago to Ann Arbor, Michigan, where her son, a musician, was giving a concert. With the support of others in the class, Barbara planned out her trip in great detail. Because she was not strong enough to carry a heavy suitcase, Barbara traveled light and wore a layered mix-and-match outfit that would last all weekend, instead of packing several outfits. She packed her toiletries in small, lightweight containers so they wouldn't weigh her down, and she called ahead to the train station for help getting on and off the train. As a result, Barbara made the trip without a hitch. More remarkably, she since has gone on to start her own consulting business, which involves international travel! "In other words, unlimited possibilities becomes the name of the game," says Connell.

Dr. Lorish says everyone can develop a more positive, can-do attitude. Here's what he suggests.

Take action. Get involved in some activity that will build your confidence and give you a taste of success. Join a water exercise class or a walking club, or take some college courses, for example. "To experience success, you've got to take action," says Dr. Lorish. "You can't just lie on your bed and daydream. You've got to get out and do it."

Fantasize about something you've given up because of arthritis but would love to do again. In Karen Connell's program, for example, one man with osteoarthritis dreamed of ballroom dancing once again—and did it. Another woman had a much humbler fantasy—to be able to bend over to clean out the vegetable bins in her refrigerator. She, too, accomplished her fantasy.

Break your goal down into smaller tasks. If you want to play golf again, for example, one mini-goal might be doing hand exercises to develop the strength to hold a golf club. Another would be walking daily to build your stamina for getting around the golf course. Think creatively, visualizing each aspect of an activity to separate out its smaller, doable components. (As a well-known Chinese proverb says, "A journey of a thousand miles must begin with a single step.")

Look to others for inspiration. Seek out people with arthritis who, despite their disabilities, have gone on to accomplish remarkable achievements. Share your plans with others and ask for suggestions. One way to meet resourceful folks with arthritis is through the Arthritis Foundation, which sponsors many different programs. (Call your local chapter for details.)

Take credit for your accomplishments and feel empowered by your achievements. "Remember that you're achieving things not through magic or luck but through your own efforts," says Dr. Lorish. The Chicago woman who finally cleaned out her vegetable bins was just as delighted with her achievement as the man who resumed ballroom dancing, says Connell.

Stress Control for Achy Joints

It's 5:30 P.M. on Friday. You're eager to get home to prepare dinner for guests, but you're stuck in a massive traffic jam. Some jerk behind you keeps honking his horn. You gnash your teeth and grip the steering wheel. Then the unthinkable happens. Your engine sputters and dies, leaving you stranded on a crowded expressway. Now you've got an even bigger problem: You're stuck, with a capital S.

If you have arthritis, hassles like these can heat up your painful joints as well as your temper. "Stress doesn't cause arthritis, but there's no question that it can aggravate arthritis," says Daniel J. Wallace, M.D., clinical assistant professor of medicine at the UCLA School of Medicine. The degree to which stress affects arthritis varies from person to person and also depends on what kind of arthritis you have, says Dr. Wallace. In general, stress is most likely to affect people with lupus, RA, and fibromyalgia. Stress also plays a minor role in aggravating osteoarthritis, he says. (Physical stress can also affect gout.)

Stress takes its toll on tender joints in several ways. As we explained in chapter 10, "The Three Rs: Relaxation, Rest, and Relief," when you're under stress, your muscles can become tight and tense. Tense muscles alone can cause pain by nudging against nerve endings or by putting pressure on sore joints. Stress also can disturb the immune system, triggering flare-ups in people with autoimmune forms of arthritis like lupus and RA, says Dr. Wallace. Finally, stress can rob you of restful sleep, which may worsen your arthritis pain during the day.

For years, doctors have noticed that people with RA often develop their initial symptoms following a major stressful event, such as the death of a loved one, an illness in the family, a divorce, or a financial crisis. "One of my patients developed symptoms three days after her son committed suicide," writes rheumatologist Warren A. Katz, M.D., in *Rheumatic Diseases: Diagnosis and Management,* a textbook on arthritis. "Another noted significant joint pain for the first time in her life after she saw her husband return from the operating room, where a brain tumor was [removed]."

Often, however, it's not a single tragedy that causes stress but an accumulation of smaller nuisances and annoyances. One researcher asked a group of patients with RA to fill out a questionnaire about their "daily hassles"—the irritations and frustrations encountered in everyday life. Each person checked off his or her pet peeves on a lengthy list of hassles, ranging from concerns about owing money to silly practical mistakes, such as misplacing a set of car keys. The results showed that people who had the greatest number of daily hassles also had the sorest, most inflamed joints and the worst morning stiffness and fatigue.

All stress isn't bad, though. Sometimes stress comes from a positive experience, such as planning your daughter's wedding, going on vacation, or falling in love. And without any stress whatsoever, life would be dreadfully dull. One researcher compares stress to the tension on a violin string: With the right tension, you can make beautiful music. With too much tension, the string snaps. As pioneer stress researcher Hans Selye, M.D., once said, "Complete freedom from stress is death."

Fight, Flight—or Flow

Strictly speaking, stress is the way the body responds to any challenging or threatening situation. Confronted with a stressful event, the body starts to churn out adrenaline and other powerful hormones. These hormones quicken the heart rate, increase blood pressure, tense the muscles, and turn on a host of other physiological responses. Thus prepared, you stand ready to either face a stressful situation or run away from it.

The trouble is, this primitive "fight or flight" response may have worked well for cave dwellers, who needed to decide in an instant whether to club a marauding bear or run for the hills. But in modern society, where the only angry bear you're likely to face is your boss, it's rarely appropriate to fight or flee. So instead, you sit and fume. Your body stews in a bath of stress hormones, with no way to diffuse the tension you've generated. For many people, the consequence is a host of physical ailments, such as stomach ulcers, headaches, and possibly, more frequent arthritis episodes. (See "The Signs of Stress" on page 171 for a checklist of symptoms commonly triggered by too much stress.)

To manage everyday tension, you need to learn and practice stress-management techniques, says Beth Ziebell, Ph.D., a psychologist in Tucson, Arizona, who has taught stress management to many arthritis patients. Here are nine steps to help you minimize stress and its effects.

Identify the sources of stress in your life. Keep a stress diary for a few days, suggests Dr. Ziebell. As you go through each day, jot down any stressful incidents, the time they occur, and any related physical symptoms. Note any connection between stress levels and your arthritis pain or other physical problems. For many people, seeing this connection is all it takes to motivate them to practice stress management, says Dr. Ziebell.

Take steps to avoid or deal with stressful events.

The Signs of Stress

Stress can cause a wide array of physical symptoms. Among the most common are:

- Anxiety.
- Change in appetite (increase or decrease).
- Cold, sweaty hands.
- Indigestion.
- General body complaints, such as headache, stomachache, or pain in the back or muscles.
- Grinding teeth or clenching jaws.
- Muscle tension.
- Nervousness, trembling.
- Sleeplessness.
- Tiredness or exhaustion.

Some of these symptoms may also be caused by other ailments. If you experience any of these signs for more than a week, talk to your doctor to determine the cause.

Once you know what causes stress, you may be able to avoid the problem. If driving to and from work at rush hour makes you tense, for example, look into the possibility of joining a van pool or taking a bus. If you can't change a stressful situation, work on responding to the problem with a more relaxed attitude. Remember, it's not the event that causes stress, but how you react to it. (Cardiologist Robert Eliot, M.D., once said, "Don't sweat the small stuff. And remember, it's almost all small stuff.")

Build natural stress-reducers into your day. Try to practice relaxation exercises twice daily. If you don't have time for a relaxation break, stop to take a few deep breaths or get up and stretch, suggests Dr. Ziebell. Shoulder shrugs also help to relieve muscle tension. Simply push your shoulders up toward your ears, hold a few seconds, then relax. Repeat several times. Daily exercise, such as swimming, bicycling, and walking, also helps to release tension. (Other relaxation techniques are discussed in chapter 10, "The Three Rs: Relaxation, Rest, and Relief.")

Be good to yourself.   Make time every day for at least one enjoyable leisure activity, no matter how small. Meet a friend for lunch, get out your sketch pad, or plant a pot of herbs. "The more harried you get, the more you need to plan some activity into your day that is pleasurable," says Dr. Ziebell. You might also splurge now and then by taking the whole day off. Kathleen Kennedy, who has fibromyalgia and osteoarthritis, tries to reduce stress in her life because it aggravates the fibromyalgia. Once in a while, she goofs off and holds a "Be-Good-to-Kathleen Day." "I might watch the soaps, daydream, or fix a photo album," she says. "The idea is to do something enjoyable I've been putting off."

Work on expressing yourself to others.   "We all know how to talk, but it's not always easy to make ourselves understood or to understand other people," says Dr. Ziebell. "Poor communication is a very high source of stress." Assertiveness, she says, is a skill most people need to improve. Learn to say no when someone asks you to do something that causes you to feel stressed or diverts you from a more important activity. Also, work on communicating anger and other negative feelings in a blame-free way. If you're angry at your kids, for example, it's better to say "I'm feeling angry about this situation," than "You're selfish and inconsiderate." Stating your feelings without blaming others helps you to discuss problems openly without hurting others' feelings and generating even more stress.

Plan ahead for particularly stressful times.   If you foresee busy times in the weeks ahead, try to space out the stressful events rather than clustering them all in one day. Use the same principle to plan each day. If you know your afternoon is going to be hectic, for example, leave your evening free for something fun and relaxing.

Be flexible.   Trying to be perfect is admirable, but unless you happen to be an angel in disguise, you're going to make your share of mistakes and blunders. Striving to be the ideal parent, employee, or boss can be very stressful. So forget it. Be content with your best effort, even if the results are less than perfect.

Don't lose your sense of humor. A good laugh is a wonderful way to dissolve tension and lighten your perspective. (For tips on brightening your life with humor, see "Getting the Last Laugh on Arthritis" on page 174.)

Don't rely on tranquilizers, alcohol, or cigarettes. These substances won't help you control stress. In fact, they can create problems—and more stress—of their own. If you're a heavy drinker or tend to abuse recreational drugs, seek professional guidance, recommends Dr. Ziebell.

Frustrated by Stiff, Achy Joints? Read This

While everybody feels blue now and then, people with serious forms of arthritis, such as RA, are more likely to be depressed than the average person. A study conducted by researchers at the University of Missouri Multipurpose Arthritis Center found that 42 percent of a group of patients with RA suffered from depression. Besides leaving you sad and gloomy, depression also can affect your sleep habits, appetite, thinking, and sex life. (If you suspect you're depressed, check your symptoms against the list in "Are You Depressed?" on page 176.)

Most people with arthritis who feel depressed have what's called reactive depression. That is, their sadness is not a mysterious deep-seated condition but an understandable reaction to a stressful or unhappy life event, such as the pain, disability, and personal loss caused by their illness. One man who had always prided himself on being the family breadwinner, for example, became depressed when he developed arthritis and had to quit his job and live on disability payments. A young mother with arthritis felt depressed because she lacked the energy to take care of her children.

"Arthritis is frustrating because you can't do all the things you used to do," says Dorothy Withrow, who has RA. "It takes twice as long to do half as much, and some things you can't do at all. You get periods of depression just because you're so frustrated."

(continued on page 176)

Getting the Last Laugh on Arthritis

Can a chuckle a day keep your arthritis pain away? Dorothy Withrow thinks so. She frequently escapes from rheumatoid arthritis pain by laughing with friends or at television comedy and game shows. "I firmly believe that laughter is good medicine," she says. "If I can find something that makes me laugh, I find that helps me to forget my pain."

Plenty of doctors agree with her. Laughter gives the muscles in the chest, abdomen, and face a good workout, helping to relieve tension and stress, according to Bernard S. Siegel, M.D., author of *Love, Medicine, and Miracles*. "Physiologists have found that muscle relaxation and anxiety cannot exist together, and the relaxation response after a good laugh has been measured as lasting as long as 45 minutes," he writes. Some studies also suggest that hearty laughter triggers the release of endorphins, the body's natural painkillers, along with other substances that fight inflammation.

Perhaps no one knows the healing power of laughter for arthritis better than Norman Cousins. A few years ago, the former *Saturday Review* editor developed ankylosing spondylitis, a chronic form of inflammatory arthritis that attacks the spine. At first, Cousins didn't see much humor in his painful condition. "Nothing is less funny than being flat on your back with all the bones in your spine and joints hurting," he recalls in his personal account, *Anatomy of an Illness*. But Cousins had the last laugh. Remarkably, he fully recovered from his disease, a recovery that he credits, in part, to laughing at "Candid Camera" reruns and old Marx Brothers films. Just 10 minutes of genuine belly laughter had an anesthetic effect and gave him at least 2 hours of pain-free sleep, he says. After each laugh session, tests also showed his inflammation subsided a bit.

Even if you've blown the punch line to every joke you've ever tried to tell, you can still brighten your life with laughter. Like any skill, your sense of humor can improve with practice, says Joel Goodman, Ed.D., director of the HUMOR Project at the Saratoga Institute in Saratoga Springs, New York. ("And humor is safer than most medications," quips one physician.) Here's how to get your funny bone in shape.

Take a humor break each day. Watch a zany television show, read a book by a humorist, or check out some comedy albums from your local library. Watching young children play is often amusing, as are the antics of a family dog or cat. The best place to find humor is in the world right around you, says Dr. Goodman.

174

Learn to laugh at yourself. "Take your job seriously but yourself lightly," says Dr. Goodman. "Tell a joke on yourself, or diffuse an embarrassing situation through humor." Howard MacDonald, for example, is not above making light of his arthritis to family and friends.

Put a humorous quotation or cartoon on your refrigerator door or the bulletin board at work. Wear a T-shirt or button with a funny message. Send a friend a greeting card with an appropriate punch line.

Put together a humor first aid kit. Fill it with the things that make you laugh: an absurd mask or wig, a silly toy, a book of cartoons, a cassette recording of your favorite comedian and a portable tape player, or some amusing photographs of you and your companions. Dig it out when life gets a little too serious.

Call or get together with friends who have a good sense of humor. Dorothy Withrow likes to laugh herself silly by getting together with her old chums from college. Twice a year, the group goes to the mountains for a few days to reminisce and share funny experiences. "We laugh all the time," she says. "No matter how bad I'm feeling, when I come home I feel great."

Memorize a funny joke or story, then wait for the right moment to share it. Dr. Goodman got a lot of "smileage" from this witty remark by Robert Frost: "The brain is a wonderful organ. It starts the moment you get up in the morning and does not stop until you get to the office!" Dr. Goodman once kept a joke-a-day calendar on his desk, which provided a ready source of humorous material.

When you hear a funny joke or story, write it down immediately. Then tell it to someone to help you remember it. But remember to use humor as a tool to make people feel good, not as a weapon to tear them down, says Dr. Goodman. Avoid jokes that are racist, sexist, or in any way offensive or mean, he says.

Be open to new kinds of humor. Pick up an album or cassette tape of a humorist you've never listened to before. Watch a movie of a comedian who's new to you. Learning to laugh at an unfamiliar style of humor—satire, slapstick, "Saturday Night Live"—is comparable to a kid eating spinach for the first time, says Dr. Goodman. If you try it, you might like it. And that's no joke.

Are You Depressed?

Depression can masquerade as many different symptoms, disrupting your thoughts, emotions, and behavior. Among the possible signs are:

- Agitation or increased activity.
- Changes in appetite.
- Decreased sex drive.
- Difficulty thinking or concentrating.
- Feelings of sadness, hopelessness, worthlessness, guilt, or self-reproach.
- Loss of interest or pleasure in daily activities.
- Shifts in sleep habits, especially waking up in the early morning before your normal rising time.
- Sluggishness, lack of energy.
- Thoughts of death or suicide.
- Weight gain or loss (unintentional).

Occasionally, depression occurs as a side effect of corticosteroid therapy, sometimes used to treat RA and lupus. (Blood pressure medications can also trigger depression.) If you use corticosteroids and feel depressed or unusually moody, ask your doctor if your depression might stem from an adverse drug reaction.

Banish the Blues

If you feel depressed, it's important to realize that you may be able to control how you feel, emphasizes Dr. Ziebell. "There may be reasons why you feel depressed—you hurt, you're disabled, or you can't do all the things you used to. Understandable as that may be, though, your depression is not inevitable. You can do something about it," she says.

One of Dr. Ziebell's favorite stories is about a 50-year-old man with RA who was severely depressed. Asked by his therapist what he really wanted to do in life, the man replied that he wanted to drive to a nearby mountain and look at the tall green trees. Strangely enough, the man could drive and was able to get to the mountain easily. Yet he hadn't made this trip in more than two years. The therapist recommended that his client take the trip that very week, and the man did. Almost instantly, his depression lifted.

The moral of this story isn't that mountain scenery is a sure cure for depression. The point is that the man snapped out of his slump simply by taking some kind of action. "Most people who are depressed do practically nothing," says Dr. Ziebell. "The first thing I ask depressed people to do is to act as if they're not depressed. Often, the very act of doing something makes them feel better."

The suggestions below, recommended by Dr. Ziebell and other therapists, may help to restore your spirits. If your depression continues for more than two weeks, consult your doctor, who may suggest counseling or antidepressant drugs. And if you have any suicidal thoughts, share your feelings right away with someone you respect, such as your doctor, a counselor, a close friend, or a clergyman.

Sort out your troubles. As we mentioned earlier, when Kathleen Lewis feels depressed, she sometimes throws a "pity party" for herself, where she sobs and really lets her emotions out. Once she has vented her sad feelings, she is able to think much more clearly and calmly about what's bothering her. She also keeps a prayer journal, where she records her thoughts in the form of a prayer. Lewis says that writing things down helps her to focus her thoughts and to find creative solutions for problems that depress her.

Think positively. Some psychologists say that if you think dark thoughts, your mood will turn gloomy and somber as well. What's more, your pessimistic thoughts may be based on false reasoning, getting you down for no good reason. A person might think, for example, "I can't do a darn thing now that I have arthritis." But a more accurate statement might be, "It's true that I can no longer take long walks, but I can go swimming, go to the movies with my friends, and learn a foreign language."

This approach to depression is called cognitive therapy, which basically involves learning to replace pessimistic self-talk with more positive self-talk, which in turn helps to rid you of depression. Cognitive therapy often works very well for people with arthritis, says Stephen Wegener, Ph.D., a clinical psychologist at the University of Virginia in Charlottesville. (A psychotherapist can teach you more about cognitive therapy.)

Force yourself to be more active. If you've given up your old activities because of arthritis, try to find new outlets and interests. If you no longer work, for example, you might volunteer for a neighborhood organization. If you can't play softball or some other sport the way you used to, maybe you can coach a team instead. If you are very limited by arthritis, consult an occupational or physical therapist, who can suggest adaptive aids to help you get around better, says Dr. Ziebell.

Discuss your feelings with someone. Kathleen Kennedy became depressed while caring for her elderly, ailing mother. "The only way I could shake off my depression was to talk to my one sister, to whom I feel very close," she says. "She was my confidante, she was the listener I needed." Aside from a friend or family member, you can also find supportive people at an arthritis self-help group. Your local chapter of the Arthritis Foundation can give you information on groups in your area.

Exercise regularly, if you can. Bicycling, walking, swimming, and other forms of exercise can lift your spirits in several ways. Regular exercise triggers the release of endorphins, natural mood-enhancing chemicals. More important, exercise gives you a psychological lift. "Exercise restores your sense of self-worth and of being somebody who is competent and capable," says Mary E. Moore, M.D., Ph.D., director of the Einstein-Moss Rehabilitation Center and professor of medicine at the Temple University School of Medicine.

Associate with upbeat people. Seek out people who make you laugh and are fun to be around. Invite them over for coffee or just call to ask how they are and what they're up to. Try to stay away from chronic complainers or cynics, at least until you feel better.

Beat Fatigue

Everyone experiences occasional fatigue when they have too much to do or not enough sleep (or both), but some people with arthritis are tired all the time. If you have active RA or lupus, for example, you may feel exhausted because your body is using all its energy to deal with inflammation. "And with any kind of arthritis, if you've been fighting pain for a long time, you can get very tired," says Cynthia Stabenow Kulp, a registered occupational therapist and instructor in the Division of Rheumatology at the University of Virginia Medical Center in Charlottesville. And if you're battling stress, depression, or insomnia, you may also lack your usual spunk.

Arthritis-related fatigue is a particularly distressing problem for people who were once real live wires. Before Howard MacDonald developed RA, for example, he says, "On a typical Saturday, I'd cut the lawn, trim the bushes, play 18 holes of golf, and then go out dancing at night. But I can't do that anymore." Now, MacDonald is careful to rest frequently and spend his limited energy wisely. "Fatigue is worse than stress," he says. "You ache, you're tired, you have no ambition or energy. You feel like everything is a burden weighing on your shoulders."

If your personal supply of go-power runs low before the day is over, try practicing some personal energy conservation. Learn new ways of doing everyday activities that help you have less pain—and more pep.

Taking your arthritis medication helps indirectly, by reducing pain and inflammation. Improving your sleep habits also may help. (For tips on restful sleep, see chapter 10, "The Three Rs: Relaxation, Rest, and Relief.") But you can take active steps to conserve your energy by learning to pace yourself, says Dr. Ziebell. She suggests scheduling short rests between periods of activity, in effect distributing what energy you do have throughout the day. Here's an example: One Saturday, Howard MacDonald wanted to prune his shrubs. Rather than doing the entire chore at once, he accomplished it in several short sessions alternated with frequent breaks. After he got out his garden tools, he stopped and went inside for a half hour. Refreshed, he was able to do some pruning for an hour or so, until he needed another short break.

How often you need to rest is up to you. But it's important to stop for a break *before* you feel tired, says Kulp. If you wait until you're exhausted, it may be too late, and your arthritis may flare up, she says. On days when your arthritis is bothering you, it's also wise to rest more than usual. "When I'm having a bad week, I have to lie down every afternoon," says a young mother with RA. "If I don't lie down, by 5:30 P.M. I'm tired and mean and crying and not worth being around. I need that rest to be the best mother I can be."

Many people with arthritis don't consider pacing themselves, and they suffer increased pain and fatigue as a result, says Dr. Ziebell. "When you're having a really good day, you want to wash the dog, wax the floor, go shopping, visit a sick friend, and try to do everything. It's understandable because you don't know when you're going to feel good again," she says. But if you learn to pace yourself, you can get more done than if you work straight through until you're exhausted. "I'm absolutely convinced that if you pace yourself, you'll accomplish more, because you won't get wiped out, then have to stay in bed for a couple of days," she says.

Her suggestion: To help you remember to take breaks, write the word "pacing" on a few index cards and post them in strategic locations such as your office, kitchen, and laundry room.

More Energy-Conservation Tips

Pacing is just one of many ways to help you overcome a personal energy shortage. Below are six more ways to fatigue-proof your life.

Set priorities. Look at your obligations and decide what's essential or important, and what's trivial and can be ignored. "Try to do what's really important to you, rather than trying to do it all," says Dr. Ziebell. One woman with RA, for example, decided that the most important thing in her life was to work as a counselor. But because just getting dressed in the morning tired her out, she hired a part-time aide to help her get dressed and ready for work, thereby conserving her available energy for what really counted.

Make a list of everything you normally do each day, suggests Kulp. Rate each activity on a 1-to-5 scale of its importance to you, with 1 being least important and 5 being most important. Now review your list. Are you spending your time doing what matters most to you? If not, can you eliminate some tasks or delegate them to others? Also, look to see if you're trying to do too much on any particular day. If so, try to spread out your activities over several days.

Simplify your daily routine. If it takes you half an hour to put on panty hose in the morning, try wearing a long skirt with knee-high stockings instead. If you're too stiff to fix breakfast for your kids most mornings, try setting the table and leaving out the cereal the night before, when your joints are more limber.

Streamline household chores. Cut down or eliminate ironing by wearing clothes made of wrinkle-free fabrics. Put away knickknacks that require tedious dusting. Also, use laborsaving appliances such as a microwave oven and food processor. (Other self-help devices that can protect your joints and save you energy are discussed in chapter 13, "Everyday Coping Tips.")

Sit instead of stand, when you can. Some people use a chair with wheels to do chores in the kitchen. If you have a job where you sit all day, however, you'll feel more refreshed if you get up and walk around occasionally. The idea is to avoid being stuck in one position for too long.

Ask for help when you need it. When one person in the family develops arthritis, everybody needs to pitch in and help with that person's chores, says Kulp. One woman with arthritis who prided herself on keeping her home spotless, for example, persuaded her husband to wash the dishes and enlisted her kids to help with laundry.

Preserve your health to conserve your strength. The better your overall health, the more energy you'll have. Try to eat nutritious food, exercise moderately, and keep your spirits up—in short, give your body every opportunity to stay well. "When you're in a lot of pain and really fatigued, you're apt to eat whatever is put in front of you, whether it's marshmallows or pizza," says Linda Hoover, who has RA. "And the more junk you eat, the worse you feel." If that sounds familiar to you, try cooking a large batch of a casserole or stew on days when you feel good, then freeze it in portions. You'll then have nourishing meals that can be conveniently reheated on a day when you don't feel like cooking.

CHAPTER

12

Arthritis and
Your Love Life

If you're like many people with arthritis, your love life may not be as satisfying as you'd like it to be. In one survey of people with various types of arthritis, 41 percent said the illness affected their sex lives. In another survey, 63 percent reported having sexual problems.

The number one problem is pain. Arthritis frequently attacks the knees, hips, lower back, and hands—parts of the body involved in lovemaking in various ways. As a result, many people with arthritis respond to sex with an "Ouch!" instead of an "Ahhhh."

The illness may also leave you too tired or depressed to be interested in sex. And if arthritis has deformed your joints or otherwise altered your appearance, you may no longer feel sexy and attractive.

(A few forms of arthritis sometimes cause complications that can directly affect the sex organs. Some men who have scleroderma, for example, don't have enough blood flow to the penis to sustain an erection. In such cases, the best course of action is to see a urologist, a doctor who specializes in diseases of the male urinary and genital tracts.)

Kathleen Lewis recalls the jolt to her femininity when her doctor told her never to wear high heels again. Because several forms of arthritis had affected her spine and other joints, Lewis was told to wear orthopedic shoes instead—footwear she considered ugly and unbecoming. "Going to pick out my orthopedic shoes was as depressing as going to a funeral," she recalls. "Putting them on and wearing them to a social event was even worse." Needless to say, the thought of wearing them on a date left her cold.

A sexual problem usually affects both partners in a relationship, not just the person with arthritis. If his wife has arthritis, for example, a man may worry about hurting her during sex. He may be reluctant to touch her, or he may even become impotent. Consequently, sexual dissatisfaction may prompt a husband or wife (or both) to get involved in an extramarital relationship or resort to heavy drinking. Eventually, the marriage may break up. (Some doctors say the divorce rate for people with rheumatoid arthritis, which affects mostly women, is higher than for those with any other chronic disease.)

Good News for Your Love Life

Sex doesn't have to sputter out of your life, though. In fact, a study conducted at Moss Rehabilitation Hospital in Philadelphia concluded that sex can help *relieve* arthritis. In this study, people with arthritis reported they were free from joint pain for more than 6 hours after sexual relations. Researchers speculate that sexual arousal reduces pain by stimulating the adrenal glands to produce more corticosteroid, a hormone that reduces joint inflammation and pain. Sexual activity also may trigger the release of endorphins, painkilling substances made by nerve cells.

And some people with arthritis say that when they're in love or romantically fulfilled, their joints temporarily stop bothering them. Famed heart surgeon Christiaan Barnard, for example, noticed that his RA stopped flaring up when he fell in love with a beautiful young woman named Barbara, whom he later married. "I cannot offer you any 'scientific' explanation, but I can say that meeting Barbara produced a degree of satisfaction in my life that may have put my body in better tune," he writes in his book, *Christiaan Barnard's Program for Living with Arthritis.* "Certainly for several years after the wedding, I virtually ceased to be a [rheumatoid arthritis] sufferer."

Health professionals offer many suggestions to help people with arthritis enjoy maximum pleasure and suffer minimum pain during sex.

Plan ahead for sex so you can enjoy it when you feel your best. If you have morning stiffness, for example, postpone sex until later in the day, when you feel more limber and relaxed. And save some energy for your romantic interlude by planning fewer daytime activities and making time to rest beforehand. "Most of us think that sex has to be spontaneous to be pleasurable. But preparing for sex doesn't have to diminish the experience," says Barbara J. Leo, R.N., a rheumatology nurse at Mary Imogene Bassett Hospital in Cooperstown, New York.

Take a warm bath or shower before sex to soothe and relax your body. Doing a set of range-of-motion exercises (described in chapter 7, "Loosening up: Stretching and Strengthening Exercises") may also limber you up. To minimize pain, you might take your regularly prescribed arthritis medicine about an hour before making love. Don't take tranquilizers or narcotic painkillers for this purpose, though—they can decrease your sex drive, says Mary P. Brassell, R.N., a rehabilitation arthritis clinical specialist at Moss Rehabilitation Hospital in Philadelphia.

Create a relaxing, sensuous atmosphere to help you forget about pain and focus on pleasure. Be imaginative, and create a romantic mood: Light a few candles, listen to some soft music, and enjoy a glass of wine with your mate (if alchohol does not interfere with your medicines).

Try satin sheets. According to people who have tried them, they feel luxurious, and the slippery surface makes lovemaking easier. (Most satin sheets are actually made of polyester and can be machine washed and dried.)

Use an electric blanket or electric mattress pad. Molly Burma, R.N., a rheumatology nurse clinician at Iowa Methodist Arthritis Center in Des Moines, Iowa, suggests that this will help keep you warm and relaxed in bed.

If a joint bothers you during sex, support it with a

pillow. If you're lying on your back, for example, putting a pillow under your knees can take pressure off both your knees and hips. (Remove the pillow afterward, though. Sleeping with a pillow under your knee can leave the joint frozen in a bent position.)

Experiment to find comfortable positions for intercourse. The traditional missionary position (woman on her back, man on top) may be too painful, especially for women with arthritic hips or men with arthritic arms, knees, or legs. A pamphlet published by the Arthritis Foundation, called *Living and Loving,* illustrates seven positions for intercourse that may be more comfortable alternatives for people with arthritis. To receive a free copy of this pamphlet, write or call your local chapter of the Arthritis Foundation.

It should be noted that some of the positions in the pamphlet may not be appropriate for people with artificial hips and knees. After hip replacement surgery in particular, you must avoid certain positions that might dislocate the artificial joint while the tissues are healing. With an artificial knee, you may need to use a pillow under the artificial joint to support it. (Again, be sure to remove the pillow afterward.) So if you've recently had total hip or knee replacement surgery, ask your surgeon when you can resume sexual intercourse, which positions for intercourse are safe, and which should be avoided and for how long.

Make love on a water bed to help cushion painful joints. This suggestions comes from Thomas C. Namey, M.D., a rheumatologist, associate professor of medicine, and director of the sports medicine program at the University of Tennessee Medical Center in Knoxville. One of his patients, a woman with arthritis in her back and hips, no longer enjoyed making love on a regular mattress because of pain. Switching to a water bed allowed her to enjoy sex again, says Dr. Namey. (The newer designs in water beds provide firmer support than older, high-motion models.)

Use gentle massage as a prelude to sex, if only to relax you. Take turns giving each other a massage, perhaps using talcum powder or body lotion to reduce friction. When it's your turn to be massaged, let your partner know what feels good and what's uncomfortable. "When your partner's hand gets near a painful area of your body, simply redirect it toward where you enjoy the touch most," advise the authors of *Living and Loving.* "Continue to share your feelings through words."

If necessary, use a water-soluble lubricant such as K-Y Jelly or Today Personal Lubricant to lubricate the vagina before intercourse. For some women, arthritis is accompanied by Sjögren's syndrome, which causes dryness of the mucous membranes around the eyes, mouth, and vagina. For severe dryness, Leslie R. Schover, Ph.D., head of the Section of Psychosexual Disorders at the Cleveland Clinic Foundation in Cleveland, recommends a suppository lubricant called Lubrin. These products are available without a prescription in drugstores. (Never use petroleum jelly for vaginal lubrication, however. It leaves you more vulnerable to infections.)

Talking to Your Mate

Sometimes arthritis is a convenient excuse for a flagging sex life. One young woman consulted her doctor about RA, which was bothering her hip. When the doctor asked about her sex life, the woman burst into tears. Although she was newly married, she confided that her husband was losing interest in her. She thought her arthritis was to blame. Sometimes her husband told her he didn't want to have sex because he didn't want to hurt her. Other times he didn't say anything; he just didn't come near her. They were drifting apart.

As it turned out, the couple did have a problem, but it had nothing to do with arthritis. When the doctor got the couple together to talk, the truth came out. The husband was an ambitious businessman who worked long hours. When he came home from work, he was too exhausted for sex. But rather than admit he was too tired to make love, he used his wife's arthritis as an excuse. As husband and wife began to talk more honestly about their feelings, they were able to solve their problem.

Good communication is the cornerstone of a happy sexual relationship, but unfortunately, many couples, like the pair in the story above, don't talk to each other about sex. "A lot of sexual problems are really compounded by poor communication," says Dr. Schover.

Dr. Namey agrees. He sometimes sees patients who wrongly blame their sexual problems on arthritis when a lack of communication is the real culprit. "Many people who have a sexual problem use their arthritis as a scapegoat," he says. "It's easier to blame your aching hip or back for your lack of desire than it is to say to your spouse, 'You never talk to me,' or 'I'm bored with our sexual routine.' "

Sexual openness is also important in cases where arthritis *is* the cause of a sexual problem. If you have pain or discomfort during lovemaking, for example, don't expect your partner to guess you're uncomfortable. "The person with arthritis may be in pain and uncomfortable, and the spouse may not be clear how to deal with it," says Barbara Leo. "If there are open lines of communication, you can avoid many sexual problems." Words will express your feelings more clearly than sighs and groans (which may be mistaken for cries of pleasure).

To help you develop more sexual openness with your partner, Dr. Schover offers some suggestions.

• Set aside some time to talk to your partner about your sex life. You might say something like, "I know it's not always easy to talk about sex, but since I've had arthritis, our love life isn't what it used to be. Let's talk about it, so we can find a way to make it better."

• Plan to talk about sex when the two of you feel relaxed and won't be disturbed. Often, the bedroom is the *last* place to talk about sex, says Dr. Schover. Choose a setting where you and your partner have held other thoughtful and intimate conversations, such as over a Sunday brunch or after dinner in the evening.

• If you would like your partner to change his or her lovemaking techniques, request just one change at a time. Too many demands, all at once, may overwhelm your mate. Trying a new position is a good start, for example.

• Be positive. Let your partner know how much you appreciate his or her willingness to make changes. When the two of you talk about your sexual relationship, don't be afraid to reveal some of your own fears and vulnerabilities, rather than dwelling solely on your partner's shortcomings. And if you enjoy a new element in your lovemaking, be sure to let your partner know how you feel.

Talking to Your Doctor about a Sexual Problem

Don't be shy about telling your doctor about a sexual problem. "Your doctor understands your disease from a medical viewpoint and is in a position to help you or to refer you to someone for counseling," says Dr. Namey. As with men who have scleroderma and fail to sustain an erection, the problem may be purely physical. And don't wait for your doctor to ask you about a sexual problem—because you may wait forever, says Dr. Schover. Although many rheumatologists routinely ask patients about their sex lives, others may overlook the subject or feel awkward bringing it up.

Here are some tips from Dr. Schover to help you discuss a sexual problem with your doctor.

• Start by saying something like, "I know you are really pressed for time, Doctor, but I'm having a problem with my sex life, and I wondered if you could give me some advice or suggest someone else who could."

• Be specific. For example: "Doctor, when my husband and I make love, my hips usually hurt, especially when we use the missionary position. Sometimes, the pain lasts as long as an hour after sex."

• Be prepared. Before your appointment, jot down some notes about the problem, such as when you first noticed the trouble, how often and when it occurs, and ways you've tried to solve it on your own.

• Be assertive. "All too often, doctors and nurses will dismiss a sexual problem or won't give you the answers you're looking for," says Dr. Schover. "You have to be prepared to deal with that, and to respond by saying, 'Well, my sex life is important to me, and if you can't help, who would you suggest I talk to?' "

Sometimes people find it easier to talk about a sexual problem with a medical social worker, an occupational therapist, or a physical therapist. These health professionals sometimes can suggest ways to cope with an arthritis-related sexual problem. If they can't help, they should refer you to someone who can. A woman can also ask her gynecologist about a sexual problem, if she prefers, says Dr. Namey. If the sexual problem is arthritis-related, the gynecologist may want to consult with your rheumatologist before offering advice on what to do.

A variety of other experts are available, too. If arthritis is stressing your marriage, for example, a marriage counselor or psychologist may help. If your doctor can't recommend a counselor, call your local chapter of the Arthritis Foundation and ask for information about anyone trained to counsel people with arthritis about their sexual problems. Or call a nearby medical school to ask if it has a sexual dysfunction clinic or a qualified sex therapist on staff, says Dr. Schover. If so, ask if they have experience treating people with arthritis or chronic diseases. You also may be able to locate a sex therapist by calling the departments of psychiatry, urology, or gynecology, she says.

Taking Arthritis on a Date

If you're single, should you tell someone you're dating about your arthritis? If so, when? And how much should you say about your illness? What if your date asks you to participate in an activity you don't feel up to? Those are just a few of the questions that can turn the dating game into a round of Twenty Questions for single people with arthritis.

As for when to tell someone about your arthritis, the answer is easy: When you're good and ready. "It's up to you whether or not to tell someone you have arthritis," says Mary Brassell. "If you can't disco until 4:00 A.M., you can either tell your date it's because of your arthritis or you can say you hurt your ankle playing tennis.

Do whatever you're comfortable with. How much you want to tell people about a health problem is entirely up to you."

Being asked out on a date that would tax your physical capabilities can be awkward, too. "These days, people are expected to be into fitness—exercising, playing tennis," says Molly Burma, who's single and has RA. "But if you've got a bad case of rheumatoid arthritis, it's hard to participate in some activities." Burma suggests talking to an occupational therapist about ways to adapt a recreational activity to your abilities. If you want to play tennis, for example, a therapist might suggest wearing a wrist splint, using a lightweight racquet, or playing doubles so you don't have to play as hard. Or you can suggest an alternate activity: If tennis is completely out of the question, ask your date if you could go to a concert or see a movie instead.

If arthritis taxes your energy levels, you may be tempted to stay home rather than get out to meet new people. Don't give in. But do allow yourself some time to rest during the day so you'll have energy for socializing. Also, try to choose social activities that help you meet people but are not too demanding. One woman with RA met her new boyfriend while taking an evening course at a local college, for example. Burma found a compatible mate through a dating service. Church social groups and volunteer organizations also can be good places to meet new people. In some cities, local chapters of the Arthritis Foundation offer support groups for young adults.

Arthritis need not automaticlly consign you to celibacy. With a little thought and consideration, you can enjoy a full, satisfying relationship with a loving partner.

13

Everyday Coping Tips

Painful arthritis doesn't keep Cynthia Brown from growing a large vegetable and flower garden every year. Thanks to an inventive aid, she can tend her plants without tiring or putting excess strain on her joints. Brown, 61, gardens while sitting on a cushion in a child's red wagon.

While traveling alone, Kathleen Ernst encountered a problem common to many with rheumatoid arthritis (RA) in their hands. She couldn't turn the key to unlock her hotel room door because her fingers were too stiff. With innovative thinking, Ernst solved her problem: The next day, she bought needle-nosed pliers. The pliers held the key, and she held the pliers. Then it was *easy* to insert the key in the lock and turn it to open the door.

Howard MacDonald, who also has RA, has trouble bending over to put on his shoes. For a few dollars, he bought a shoehorn with a handle 2 feet long, which allows him to slip his shoes on easily and without strain.

Like these three people, you can find helpful gadgets to make living with arthritis easier and more comfortable. With the aid of self-help devices, you can dress, cook dinner, drive a car, and enjoy most other activities with minimal stress and strain. (Self-help, of course, doesn't *always* mean reaching for a gadget. Sometimes all you need to do is think of simpler ways to do things, like sitting down to garden or asking someone to give you a hand with a heavy bag of groceries.)

People with arthritis are ingenious: They've found dozens of coping tips to help outsmart the disease. Occupational therapists, too, can often suggest devices for specific problems, show you how to use them, and steer you to retail stores or mail-order catalogs that sell them.

The devices described in this chapter are available at most medical supply stores. Or you can order them from the mail-order catalogs listed in "Resource Guide for Self-Help Aids and Services" on page 206. You can make some devices at home, using materials such as Velcro or foam rubber. Others, like a garden seat, can be adapted from things you may already own. You can pick and choose among the various ideas presented here, adopting those that work best for you.

Don't underestimate the role of self-help aids in relieving arthritis. The right tool or technique can prevent pain, save you energy, and even stop a vulnerable joint from becoming deformed, says Evelyn Rossky, a retired rheumatology therapist who worked with arthritis patients for many years at Moss Rehabilitation Hospital in Philadelphia. What's more, she says you should use the aids routinely, even on days when your joints don't hurt, to help protect them from wear and tear. (*Editor's Note:* One rheumatologist we spoke to cautions that not everyone agrees that using self-help aids can prevent deformity; this is controversial.)

Coping Tips around the House

Ahh, home sweet home—unless your stairs are impossible to climb, or you have to stretch and strain to reach the kitchen cabinets. For many with arthritis, a house can seem like an obstacle course. An overstuffed sofa or chair, for instance, may look like an inviting place to sit down. Trying to get up again is another matter. And electric appliances are no convenience if you can't turn the control knobs.

If arthritis leaves you feeling helpless in your own home, it's time to declare your independence. Here are some suggestions to help you cope with common problems around the house.

Knob grippers. If arthritis affects your hands, it may be hard to turn doorknobs, water faucets, and stove controls. Knob-turning devices in various shapes to fit a variety of household knobs are available from retailers listed in the resource guide on page 206. Most have a rubber cup that grips the knob and a handle that you press to turn it.

Needle-nosed pliers. If you have trouble grasping small objects, try using this versatile household gadget, says Rossky. Besides using them to grip door keys, you can use the pliers to turn some appliance knobs, open soda cans that have pull tabs, or pull belt ends through buckles.

Reacher. If you can't bend or reach easily, you can use a long-handled device called a reacher, which has a pair of tongs on one end. It allows you to pick up small items from the floor or in tall cabinets and shelves. When you squeeze the handle, the tongs grip the object you want to pick up. Some reachers have a magnet on the end to make it easier to pick up small metal objects such as keys.

Telephone aids. Since dialing a telephone can be a difficult task for arthritic fingers, use a pencil to turn a rotary dial or to depress the digits on a push-button phone. If holding a telephone receiver bothers your neck or arms, have a speaker phone hooked up.

Pencil grippers. To grip a pen or pencil more easily, enlarge it with a foam hair curler. And a felt-tip pen may be easier to use than a ballpoint, because you don't have to press as hard.

Self-opening scissors. If cutting paper or fabric is difficult, try using a pair of lightweight self-opening scissors. A spring opens them automatically after each cut. Self-opening scissors reduce thumb strain and make cutting almost effortless.

Light-switch extender. If you can't reach up to turn a light switch on and off, install a light-switch extension handle. The long handle puts the light's toggle switch within easy reach of people in wheelchairs or those with limited arm movement.

Stair-climbing aids. For many people with arthritis in the hips and knees, climbing stairs is a real challenge. To provide two-handed support, mount a rail or bannister on both sides of the stairwell. To make the job easier still, climb stairs one at a time,

(continued on page 196)

No-Fuss Cooking Tips

Does cooking feel like a Herculean task, especially on days when your joints are acting up? With planning and few shortcuts, you can whiz through kitchen duty with minimal stress on your joints—and on you. Think of cooking as an investment in your health. By putting small amounts of time and energy into making wholesome meals, you'll reap the dividends of better nutrition.

Keep these helpful hints in mind.

1. Plan ahead. Minimize last-minute distress by deciding what meals you want to make for the week ahead and what ingredients you'll need. Double or triple a recipe, then freeze the leftovers for an easy meal another day. Soups, stews, and casseroles freeze especially well.

2. Delegate. Let other family members pitch in with cooking. Or when you shop, ask a friend or neighbor to help you carry groceries inside and put them away.

3. Zip through grocery shopping. If you arrange your shopping lists according to where items are in the store, you'll get done faster. It helps if you usually shop in the same place and know the store layout.

4. Use lightweight pots and pans. Forget heavy iron skillets—coated nonstick aluminum pans are much lighter. Also, use plastic or stainless steel bowls instead of ceramic bowls or crockery.

5. Lift the food, not the pot. Instead of struggling with heavy colanders of food, use a wire-mesh strainer to remove spaghetti or vegetables from a large pot.

6. Avoid battles with stuck-on food by broiling in disposable aluminum pans.

7. Stabilize mixing bowls by setting them on a damp cloth or piece of nonskid plastic.

8. Sit to prepare meals. Get a chair with good back support that adjusts in height. Consider one with wheels so you can push yourself around the kitchen.

9. Keep items that you use often, such as flour, sugar, and spices, on the counter rather than in hard-to-reach cupboards.

10. Put your meals on wheels. Use a wheeled plant stand to move heavy items, such as a stew pot, across the counter. Similarly, a rolling cart is helpful for transporting food from counter to table and back.

11. To easily open the refrigerator, tie a string loop through the handle. Slip your forearm through the loop and pull to open. The same tip works for cabinet and drawer handles.

12. To open jars, use a nubby rubber disk to give more friction. Or mount a jar opener that will grip the lid as you use both hands to open it. If you live alone, ask the checker at the grocery store to open new jars for that first difficult twist. Ask family members to cooperate by closing lids with only half a twist instead of tightly.

13. Let machines work for you. A food processor is great for chopping and slicing. A blender, a lightweight portable mixer, an electric knife, and an electric can opener also are useful.

14. If you don't have a microwave oven, consider one. It's easy to open, it cooks fast, and it creates fewer dirty dishes. You can heat food on a paper plate, the world's lightest cooking utensil.

15. Use sharp knives. A dull knife takes extra effort to cut, chop, dice, and slice food. To keep knives sharp, store them where they won't get nicked, and don't use them to cut paper or open cartons.

16. Slice foods with a pizza wheel. Its rolling motion may be easier on your hands. You may want to get the wheel professionally sharpened. A pizza wheel works best with relatively flat foods, such as sandwiches, pies, quiches, celery, and green beans.

17. Buy frozen chopped onions or green peppers rather than dicing your own. You can also buy fresh tossed salad ingredients, already washed and cut, from salad bars in most grocery stores.

18. Use mitt-type potholders to pick up hot pans with the palms of both hands, saving strain on your wrists.

19. Use long matchsticks to light a gas oven if bending over is difficult.

20. To whip sauces, always use a whisk instead of a fork—it'll take half the effort.

21. Garnish your food with a slice of pimiento, a sprig of parsley, a fresh basil leaf, or an orange slice. It'll perk up your appetite and diguise flaws if your preparation isn't picture perfect.

22. Entertain with ease. If you don't have the energy to cook for a crowd, hold a potluck dinner and let each guest bring a different dish.

resting both feet on the same step before trying the next one. If you can afford it, consider installing a home elevator or a chair lift that goes up and down the bannister.

More Laborsaving Tips

Looking for ways to save your energy while housecleaning? Here are some helpful hints.

● Consolidate all your cleaning supplies in one closet so they'll be handy when you need them.

● A lightweight electric broom is easier to use than a heavy vacuum cleaner.

● If you can't bend or reach easily, replace your regular dustpan with a long-handled model. To clean the bathtub, use a long-handled sponge mop.

● If getting out of chairs is difficult, save your overstuffed furniture for company. For an easier lift-off, choose a chair with a firm seat, a fairly straight back, and armrests. When you're sitting, your feet should rest flat on the floor. If they don't, use a footrest to support your feet.

Here's an easy and efficient way to get up from a chair, says Rossky: First, slide your buttocks forward so that your knees are over your feet. Then, lean forward so your chin lines up with your knees. With your palms pressing down on the chair arms, push off, using both your hips and knees. (If you have RA, protect your wrists by using your forearms, not your hands, to press against the chair. Alternatively, rest your forearms on a tabletop and push off.)

Maneuvering around the Bathroom

The bathroom is probably the most treacherous room in the house. Wet, slippery surfaces can cause a fall. Folks with arthritis can get stuck in a bathtub or have trouble raising themselves off a toilet seat.

To prevent mishaps, make sure your bathroom has plenty of safety features. Place a rubber mat or apply safety strips on the tub floor. To help you maneuver in the bathtub or shower, have safety rails mounted on the walls. Never hold onto a shower curtain rod or soap dish for support, cautions Barbara Cortellini-Benamy, registered occupational therapist and a clinical supervisor of the Occupational Therapy Department at Moss Rehabilitation Hospital in Philadelphia.

"Getting into and out of the bathtub can be a very tricky maneuver," adds Rossky. So a shower may be a more convenient alternative. Here are some handy aids.

Shower bench. If you can't stand for long, sit down on a shower bench or a webbed plastic lawn chair. Use a hand-held shower unit.

Transfer bench. Some people with arthritis in their legs have trouble stepping over the tub wall into the shower. To solve that problem, use a transfer bench. The bench sits with one end in the tub and the other on the bathroom floor. To get into the tub, you sit on the bench and raise your legs over the tub edge. During the shower, you sit on the bench. (To keep your bathroom floor from getting wet while you shower: Place the transfer bench over the side of the tub. Pull the shower curtain across the full length of the tub. Using scissors, cut two vertical slits in the shower curtain, to correspond with the two outermost legs of the bench. This creates a flap approximately the width and height of the bench. Tuck the shower curtain itself inside the tub and let the flap remain outside the tub.)

Soap-on-a-rope. Whether you bathe or shower, it's helpful to wear soap-on-a-rope around your neck. This bar of soap hangs like a big locket on a rope approximately 30 inches long. Using it can eliminate a slippery hunt for runaway soap.

Back scrubber. If your reach is limited, use a long-handled brush to scrub your back and other hard-to-reach areas.

Terry cloth robe. To dry yourself after showering, throw on a terry cloth robe instead of toweling dry, suggests Rossky. You might even snuggle into bed for a minute until you feel dry, warm, and relaxed, she adds.

Toilet devices. If you have trouble sitting down on or rising from the toilet, the simplest solution is a raised toilet seat. These seats, which fit on top of a regular toilet bowl, raise the sitting level an extra 4 or 5 inches. (A commode that fits over a toilet will do the same thing.) As a result, people with hip and knee problems can sit down and get up more easily. Elevated toilet seats are a big help after total hip and knee replacement surgery. For extra support, safety rails also can be mounted around the toilet. For people with limited reach, long-handled devices to use toilet paper also are available.

Getting Dressed with Ease

Beauty may be only skin-deep, but when you feel and look attractive, your morale soars. "When I'm dressed nicely, I feel like a million bucks," says one woman with RA. "I don't feel sick."

Still, tugging on socks, pulling up zippers, and fastening buttons can be a real challenge when your joints are sore and stiff. Getting dressed in the morning can be especially trying since that's the worst time of day for many people with arthritis.

To make dressing a snap, shop for clothes that are easy to get on and off, advises Rossky. For women, loose-fitting clothes of soft fabrics tend to look feminine and are the easiest to get into and move around in, she says. To find flattering, easy-to-wear styles, "window-shop" at home by looking through clothing catalogs. Several mail-order companies (listed in the resource guide on page 206) design attractive fashions for people with arthritis and other physical limitations. Write to them for catalogs.

Some possible choices include wraparound skirts and dresses, stretchy, roomy pullover tops, and sweaters and jackets with front zippers. You may want to avoid back zippers and watch out for small buttons and snaps, which can be hard to fasten. Pants and skirts with elastic waistbands usually work well, as long as you can easily stretch the waistband over your hips. Drawstring closures on shorts, slacks, and skirts make them a cinch to get on. You can sometimes add a drawstring closure to a skirt or slacks by running a piece of ribbon or seam tape through the waistband, says Rossky. Pull the ribbon ends out through a small opening on the front or side, and tie to close.

Velcro fasteners are a blessing for many people with arthritis, says Rossky. Velcro can be used to fasten shirts, pants, belts, and running shoes, and to attach bows onto dressy blouses. If you have a shirt or coat that's hard to button, it can be adapted for easier wear by adding hidden Velcro closures. (If you don't sew or if sewing is hard for you to manage, you might have a seamstress friend or a dressmaker make the alterations.) Here's how to do it: Cut off the buttons, and resew them in place on top of the buttonholes. Then sew one piece of Velcro underneath each buttonhole and another piece where each button was. (Velcro is available in most sewing stores, and press-on Velcro is also available.)

The self-help devices listed below also can help you get dressed more easily.

Button aid. If you have trouble manipulating buttons, try a button aid, which consists of a wire loop attached to a handle. Just insert the wire loop through a buttonhole, snare the button, and pull it through the buttonhole.

Zipper pull. A zipper pull is simply a metal hook on a handle. Insert the hook into the zipper tab and pull up with the handle. (You can make your own zipper pull by attaching a partly opened paper clip to a loop of string. Insert the end of the paper clip into the tab and pull up with the loop.)

Dressing stick. If you have trouble bending or reaching, a dressing stick—a long rod with a hook on one end—is helpful for pulling up pants, underwear, and other garments or retrieving clothes that are slightly out of reach. You can also use it to pull open a dresser drawer or lift a clothes hanger out of a closet.

Sock aid. To put on socks without bending over, try a sock aid. Complete directions come with the device. Aids to pull up panty hose also are available.

Elastic shoelaces. You can leave these tied and just pull on them to put on or take off your shoes.

Easy Grooming Tips

If joint stiffness or limited mobility makes personal hygiene awkward, don't despair. Here are some tips that should make grooming easier.

Hair care. If it's hard to reach every part of your do, don't—let a long-handled comb or brush handle the job. And keep combing and every other hair chore easy by choosing a cut that doesn't need a lot of special attention.

Brushing your teeth. To get a firmer grasp on a toothbrush, attach a piece of foam rubber or a commercial utensil grip to the handle. Grips are available from Fred Sammons or Maddak, Inc., listed in the resource guide on page 206. An electric toothbrush may also make brushing easier. If you have trouble flossing, buy a dental floss holder, available in many drugstores. The holder allows you to floss with one hand.

Shaving. Men with arthritis in their hands or arms may prefer electric shavers rather than hand razors. Women who have trouble reaching to shave their legs can buy depilatory creams or make long-handled shavers by taping a wooden dowel rod to a safety razor. (Duct tape or electrical tape works best; masking tape loosens when it gets wet.)

The Easy Path to Gardening

Don't let arthritis turn your green thumb a painful shade of red. By learning easier ways to garden, you can take good care of plants and your joints, says Vicki Givler, an occupational therapist who teaches "adapted gardening" techniques to people with arthritis.

"In many cases, people don't know what kinds of adapted gardening methods are available, so they give up something they truly enjoy, rather than learning new ways to continue gardening," says Givler, who works for the Arthritis-Back Rehabilitation Unit of Rheumatology Associates, an arthritis clinic in Springfield, Massachusetts.

Don't plant more than you really need. One of the biggest mistakes people make is planting a garden that's too big for their needs, she says. "By mid-July, they have so much produce, they get exhausted trying to harvest and put up the food." Her suggestion: Plant a garden that's big enough to feed your family, not the entire neighborhood!

Plan a well-spaced garden. Be sure plants are accessible from all sides, so you can reach in easily to weed or pick produce. Ideally, garden rows should be about 2 feet wide, with an adjacent walkway wide enough for a stool or garden cart.

Get off your feet. Givler advises people with arthritis to sit down to garden, which saves energy and reduces stress on the joints. Cynthia Brown, as mentioned at the beginning of the chapter, loves using a child's wagon as a garden seat. "It's much more comfortable than kneeling on the ground, and I can push myself along in the wagon," says Brown, who is one of Givler's former students. To make the seat level with the wagon, she sits on a cushion on top of a block of wood. The wagon also serves as her garden cart, where she stores small tools. When her gardening chores are finished, she pulls the wagon back to its storage site, so she has little to carry.

Look for an inexpensive but sturdy child's wagon at a flea market or discount department store, says Givler. If you have trouble rising from a low seat, look for a wagon with large wheels or raise the seat with pillows, suggests Rossky. You can also use an empty milk crate (available at department stores) or a footstool, although they won't roll, of course.

Garden scoots, which are rolling seats mounted on wheels, also are available from garden supply stores and some mail-order suppliers. Garden scoots and other gardening tools for people with physical limitations can be ordered by mail from the Gardener's Supply company. To receive a free catalog, write to Gardener's Supply, 128 Intervale Road, Burlington, VT 05401. Or call (802) 863-1700.

Here are more easy gardening ideas from Givler.

Wear an apron. A carpenter's apron can hold your seeds, small tools, and other supplies, so you don't have to bend over as often to pick things up.

Cart it. Use a garden cart or wagon to carry heavier tools and supplies, Givler advises. A garden cart is lighter and easier to use than a wheelbarrow, she adds.

Take five. Take frequent rests between gardening chores. "Pacing is easily neglected because nobody wants to lose time. But the people who take it easy feel less pain," says Givler. If you tend to get so absorbed in your work that you forget to rest for a few minutes, set a kitchen timer to go off every hour or so and keep it within earshot.

Avoid the heat. Garden early or late in the day when it's cooler so you won't get as tired.

Time-share. To cut down on gardening chores, consider sharing your garden with a friend or neighbor.

Sow with ease. If you have difficulty bending over to sow seeds, drop them to the ground through a long tube, such as the cardboard tubes used for gift wrap. Then use a long-handled tool to cover the seed with dirt. If grasping tiny seeds is a problem, buy large, pelletlike, clay-coated seeds.

Eliminate plant thinning. Plant seeds the correct distance apart for mature plants so you don't have to thin the rows later. "By eliminating this step, you save energy and make the job easier," says Givler.

Grow up. If you can't bend over to reach your plants, let them come up to meet you. Train plants to grow vertically on a trellis (a latticework frame that will support climbing plants). If properly supported, beans, peas, tomatoes, cucumbers, and even squash will grow vertically. Trellises and other vertical growing systems are available from the Gardener's Supply catalog and other garden retailers. Or make your own trellis with chicken wire or string and wood stakes.

Make your bed. Raised garden beds also allow you to grow plants with less reaching and bending. Raised beds can be made with wood, bricks, or stone walls filled with soil. If you plan to sit to garden, the raised bed should be about 2 feet high; if you want to stand, make the garden about 6 inches taller, suggests Givler. (Or try container gardening in pots placed on top of a picnic table or utility cart.)

Cover it. Cut down on weeding by generously mulching around plants. Garden clippings, leaves, straw, bark, and even newspaper work well as mulch.

Water wisely. Use a sprinkler system to water plants. Never carry heavy buckets of water, cautions Givler. "A watering system that can be set up and left in place, then turned on and off as needed, is ideal," she says.

Get a grip on it. For a more comfortable grip on gardening tools, enlarge the diameter of the handles with foam rubber. Many hardware stores sell foam pipe insulation in the shape of hollow tubes that can be slipped over tool handles. Also, wear a pair of good gardening gloves to protect your hands.

Extend yourself. Choose garden tools with extended handles to minimize reaching and bending. Long-handled tools sold by Gardener's Supply include a 30-inch weeder and a long watering wand that attaches to the garden hose. You can also lengthen the tools you already own by securely taping a broom handle or wooden dowel to the handle.

Plant laborsaving perennials. They will spring up year after year. Brown has a beautiful perennial flower garden with daffodils, tulips, phlox, tiger lilies, daisies, and chrysanthemums. Edible perennials include asparagus, rhubarb, and horseradish.

Brace yourself. If arthritis affects your wrists or hands, protect your joints by wearing wrist splints when you garden, Givler advises. Pharmacies sell wrist splints, but it's wise to check with an occupational therapist to make sure the splint is correctly positioned.

Car Comfort

Does your enthusiasm for a car trip often stall in the driveway because you can't open the car door or maneuver into the seat? Don't spin your wheels in frustration. Here's a list of driving aids to help you enjoy your car in comfort and safety. These devices are available from self-help equipment catalogs and in some cases, from auto supply stores.

Special devices are available to open either push-button or pull-up door handles more easily. Another way to open a push-button handle is to press the button with the side of your hand rather than using your thumb. Or carry a small plastic hammer in your bag to push the button if using any part of your hand would be difficult or painful. Another helpful device is a car key aid, which holds the key firmly in a small strip of metal or plastic. It gives you enough extra leverage to turn a key more easily in the door lock or ignition. Use a padded steering wheel cover, which gives a larger and more comfortable grip, if you have arthritis in your hands. Make your own cover from foam insulation or buy one made of sheepskin or leather.

If you have trouble getting out of your car, place two thin foam pads, each covered with a slippery fabric such as rayon, on the seat. The top pad will rotate over the bottom pad when you try to slide off the seat, allowing you to move with less effort. (Aids for Arthritis listed in the resource guide on page 206, sells a ready-made swivel pad for about $23.) An auto dealer may be able to install a bucket seat that will rotate from the driving position to the door, but this is costly.

To avoid fatigue, drive with adequate support for your joints. Place a rolled-up towel behind your lower back to provide back support. Support your elbow on an armrest or small pillow. To prevent stiffness on a long drive, stop occasionally and get out to stretch or walk around.

If you have difficulty turning your neck to see behind and around the car, replace your regular rearview and sideview mirrors with wide-angle ones, available in auto supply stores.

If you need to make more modifications, consult one of the 200 occupational therapists nationwide who specialize in helping disabled drivers. If your doctor doesn't know of any, call the nearest rehabilitation hospital and ask for the occupational therapy department. If its staff doesn't have an occupational therapist with this specialized skill, perhaps it can refer you to someone.

One such therapist, Carmella Strano, is director of the Department of Transportation Evaluation and Training at Moss Rehabilitation Hospital in Philadelphia. Strano tells the story of a young woman with juvenile RA who was unable to use her feet to operate the gas and brake pedals of a car. She now drives a specially designed van that is operated only with hand controls. She controls the brakes and accelerator by pulling up or depressing the steering wheel; push-buttons operate the doors, windows, turn signals, and even the horn.

Besides occupational therapists, another excellent resource for disabled drivers is a booklet called *The Handicapped Driver's Mobility Guide,* published by the American Automobile Association (AAA). The book, available for a small charge, has a state-by-state list of rehabilitation centers and auto equipment suppliers set up to help disabled drivers. To get a copy, write or call your nearest AAA chapter. Address your inquiry to either the traffic safety or the public relations office.

Travel Tips

RA hasn't kept Howard MacDonald from seeing the world. Despite his limited energy and mobility, MacDonald has visited the Aztec ruins in Mexico, cruised around the Greek Isles, gone sightseeing in Tunisia, and explored the catacombs of Rome, to name just a few of his many exciting excursions.

How does he do it? "Planning, planning, and more planning," he says. Long before each trip, Howard begins to think through all the problems he might encounter. Then he works with his trusted travel agent to tailor his plans to his physical capabilities. He books his accommodations in hotels with elevators, since he can't climb many steps. He makes sure the bathroom in his hotel has a shower with support bars. And he calls ahead to the airline to arrange for help carrying his hand luggage on and off the plane. In short, MacDonald tries to plan every detail of his trip. "If I go on a cruise, you can bet I'm going to know that ship better than the captain," he says with a smile.

If you don't have the patience for detailed planning, a number of travel agencies will gladly do the work for you. Your best bets are agencies that specialize in arranging trips for people who use wheelchairs or have other physical disabilities. (See the section, "Travel Resources for People with Arthritis," in the resource guide on page 206). "Travel can be a very enjoyable experience for people with disabilities," says Edna Cook, director of Flying Wheels Travel. Her agency arranges both group tours and independent

(continued on page 208)

Resource Guide for
Self-Help Aids and Services

The listings below will help you find many of the devices and services mentioned in this chapter.

Where to Buy Self-Help Devices
Self-help devices are available at many medical supply stores or can be ordered from these mail-order firms.

Aids for Arthritis, Inc.
3 Little Knoll Court
Medford, NJ 08055
(609) 654-6918
Free catalog.

Cleo, Inc.
3957 Mayfield Road
Cleveland, OH 44121
1-800-321-0595
Free catalog.

Maddak, Inc.
6 Industrial Road
Pequannock, NJ 07440-1993
(201) 694-0500
Free catalog.

Fred Sammons, Inc.
Dept. 400, Box 32
Brookfield, IL 60513-0032
1-800-323-5547
Free catalog; specify Enrichments for
  Better Living.

Sears, Roebuck and Co.
Customer Relations
Sears Tower
Chicago, IL 60684
(312) 875-2500
Catalog $1; specify Home Health
  Care.

Swedish Rehab
100 Spence Street
Bay Shore, NY 11706
1-800-645-5272
1-800-424-2458 (in New York)
Free catalog.

Mail-Order Sources
for Easy-to-Wear Clothing
These companies offer stylish, up-to-date clothing that's easy to get on and off.

Comfortably Yours
61 West Hunter Avenue
Maywood, NJ 07607
(201) 368-3499
Free catalog; also sells other self-help
  devices.

EASEWEAR Unlimited
44 Wexford Drive
Mendham, NJ 07945
1-800-451-9127
Catalog $1; refundable with first
  purchase.

Fashion Ease
Division of M&M Apparel Co.
1541 60th Street
Brooklyn, NY 11219
1-800-221-8929
(718) 853-6376 (in New York)
Free catalog.

Irwin/Taylor
P.O. Box 10510
Rochester, NY 14610
1-800-356-2456
Catalog $1.

Travel Resources
for People with Arthritis

These travel agencies specialize in group and individual tours for people who use wheelchairs or have other physical disabilities.

Flying Wheels Travel, Inc.
143 West Bridge
P.O. Box 382
Owatonna, MN 55060
1-800-533-0363

Wings on Wheels
Evergreen Travel Service
19505 (L) 44th Avenue W
Lynnwood, WA 98036
(206) 776-1184

Whole Person Tours, Inc.
P.O. Box 1084
Bayonne, NJ 07002
(201) 858-3400
Also publishes *Itinerary,* a travel
magazine for people with physical
disabilities.

These are information services for travelers.

International Association for Medical
Assistance to Travelers
417 Center Street
Lewiston, NY 14092
(716) 754-4883
Provides a free annual directory of
English-speaking physicians and
medical institutions worldwide. All
physicians have been trained in the
United States, Canada, or Great
Britain and have had their
qualifications reviewed and
approved by a medical board.

Society for the Advancement of Travel
for the Handicapped
26 Court Street, Suite 110
Brooklyn, NY 11242
(718) 858-5483
Serves as a resource center for
disabled travelers, providing
information on hotels, carriers, travel
destinations, and car-rental
agencies.

(continued)

Resource Guide for Self-Help Aids and Services—Continued

Travel Resources—*Continued*

Travel Information Service
Moss Rehabilitation Hospital
12th Street and Tabor Road
Philadelphia, PA 19141
(215) 456-9600

For a small fee, provides information to disabled travelers on accessible accommodations, cruises, restaurants, and travel destinations in the United States and abroad.

Consult these books and pamphlets on special travel services.

Access Amtrak
Public Affairs Office
Amtrak
400 North Capital Street NW
Washington, DC 20001
1-800-USA-RAIL
Free guidebook explains Amtrak
  services for elderly or disabled
  passengers; phone orders only.

Access Travel: Airports
Consumer Information Center
Pueblo, CO 81009
(719) 948-3334
Lists accessibility features of 472
  airports worldwide.

*Frommer's Guide for the Disabled
  Traveler: The United States, Canada,
  and Europe* by Frances Barish
(Simon & Schuster)

*Helping Hand Program for the
  Handicapped*
Greyhound Lines, Inc.
c/o Customer Service
901 Main Street, Suite 2523
Dallas, TX 75202
The program allows a handicapped
  person and a travel companion to
  travel together on a Greyhound bus
  for one fare. To qualify, the
  handicapped person needs a written
  statement from a doctor. Details are
  provided in Greyhound's free
  brochure, *A Traveler's Guide for the
  Handicapped*, available from the
  above address or at Greyhound bus
  terminals.

travel worldwide for physically handicapped customers and their friends or relatives.

To help you plan a trip, here are some suggestions to keep in mind.

- To get the best help from your agent, explain your physical limitations and whether you use a cane, walker, or wheelchair. Also, let the agent know if you have trouble climbing stairs, walking long distances, or carrying luggage in an airport, bus, or train terminals.

- Choose a hotel that's easy to get around in. Many hotels have rooms specially designed for physically disabled travelers. Usually the rooms are near elevators and have bathrooms with support bars and other adaptations for people in wheelchairs. If you use a wheelchair or have trouble climbing stairs, make sure the hotel has entrance ramps, plus elevators to all floors.

- Check with your airline to see what kind of assistance is available to help you carry luggage or board the plane. If you can't walk long distances, most domestic airlines will transport you to and from your gate in a wheelchair or electric cart. Ask about this service when you buy your ticket. You might also want to ask which of the aircraft have on-board wheelchairs, removable armrests on the aisle seats so you can slide into your seat more easily, and lavatories that are accessible to the handicapped or have handgrips.

- Pack sparingly so you have less to carry. To save space, pack toiletries in small, lightweight plastic bottles. Bring clothes that mix and match so you can vary your wardrobe with just a few articles of clothing. Lightweight nylon luggage is a good choice. So is luggage with wheels and a pull-strap or handle. Pack any self-help aids you usually use to dress or groom yourself, such as a long-handled shoehorn or dressing stick.

- Take extra medication with you. MacDonald takes twice as much medicine as he plans to use, storing half in his suitcase and carrying the rest with him. If either parcel is lost, he won't have to do without.

- Rest between sightseeing excursions. If you will arrive at your destination after a long flight or car trip, you might want to schedule a day of rest when you arrive. Similarly, if you habitually have morning stiffness, schedule activities later in the day when you feel perkier.

Medical Help
for Arthritis

14

What You Should Know about Arthritis Drugs

The story sounds like one you'd expect to read in the *National Enquirer,* not the *New England Journal of Medicine,* where it was reported. A 70-year-old woman went to her doctor with a bizarre complaint. For the past three weeks, she'd been hearing music—mostly songs from the 1930s and 1940s. The trouble is, she heard the music day and night, wherever she went, even when she sat in a soundproof room.

Was she losing her marbles? Becoming senile? Not at all. She was quite healthy, except for her rheumatoid arthritis (RA), for which she took lots of aspirin. In fact, the woman was suffering from an aspirin overdose, which was producing aural hallucinations to the tune of Benny Goodman. When her doctor cut her aspirin dosage in half, the music stopped.

The moral of the story: Too much of a good thing can drive you crazy, whether it's big band tunes or a "wonder drug" like aspirin.

But the side effects of aspirin are rarely a laughing matter. The drug can cause stomach bleeding, ulcers, and other serious problems. And if so familiar and seemingly harmless a drug as aspirin can have side effects like these, imagine what more powerful medicines can do. It's a hard pill to swallow, but it's a fact: No matter which arthritis drug you take, you need to know about its benefits *and* its risks.

Consider another story: Howard MacDonald, 68, has had RA for 25 years. In that time, MacDonald has used enough arthritis medicines to stock a hospital pharmacy. One drug sent him to the hospital for a bleeding ulcer; another gave him cataracts. Yet he says the pain relief the drugs provide is worth it. "They give me relief from my arthritis. I know the price, and I'm willing to pay it."

Positives and Negatives: Know about Both

If you have a mild case of bursitis or tendinitis, maybe all you need to keep you pain-free until the problem subsides is a single shot of steroids, two weeks of nonsteroidal anti-inflammatories (NSAIDs), or just rest and local heat. If you suffer from gout, modern drugs are so successful you need never have another flare-up. And if you have RA, powerful drugs sometimes can put your disease into remission. But drugs are rarely a *cure* for arthritis: Most treat the symptoms, not the cause, of your discomfort. And if your joints are damaged, no drug can repair them (although the right medicines may prevent future problems).

"Drugs are extremely important for symptomatic relief," says Jeffrey Lisse, M.D., assistant professor of rheumatology at the University of Texas Medical Branch, Galveston. "They're very important for day-to-day functioning, to help people live normal lives."

Taking medication is like trying to balance a scale, with a drug's therapeutic powers on one side and its side effects on the other. You can tip these scales in your favor, however. This chapter will explain how arthritis medicines can be used safely and wisely, and what side effects to watch out for.

Aspirin

Aspirin is touted as "the wonder drug that works wonders." It's supposed to deliver "fast, fast pain relief." And for many people, aspirin does just that. So it really is the drug "doctors recommend most" for many types of arthritis, including RA and osteoarthritis.

Because aspirin is such a commonplace remedy, many people are surprised when their doctors prescribe it for a serious condition like arthritis. "There's an idea in people's minds that aspirin is not a drug because you can buy it at any supermarket," says Dr. Lisse. "Patients think, 'Doctor, I just paid you $60 for an office visit and you want me to take aspirin? Give me some real medicine!' "

But aspirin *is* real medicine. One or two tablets will relieve minor aches and pains like mild headaches or muscle soreness. In higher doses—the equivalent of 12 to 18 tablets or more a day—aspirin acts as a potent anti-inflammatory drug, able to reduce swelling and stiffness as well as pain. "You can't just take headache doses of aspirin for diseases like rheumatoid arthritis," says Dr. Lisse. "Lower doses may suffice when all you need is symptomatic relief for mild cases of osteoarthritis. But only large amounts will control inflammation."

But aspirin has some major side effects—so major that if aspirin were introduced today, the Food and Drug Administration would not allow it to be sold without a prescription. Even small amounts of aspirin can be hard on the stomach, triggering excess stomach acid, breaking down the stomach's defenses against acid, and causing nausea, heartburn, loss of appetite, or bloating. Occasionally, it causes bleeding ulcers. Rarely, it can cause serious damage to the liver, kidneys, or bone marrow.

You'd think that the more aspirin you take and the longer you take it, the greater would be your risk for side effects. The fact is, however, that some people develop ulcers soon after they start to take aspirin, while many others take aspirin for years and have no problems. Some people are more vulnerable than others and should not take aspirin. Doctors rarely prescribe aspirin for people who have certain bleeding disorders, such as hemophilia, or a history of stomach ulcers, for example. Still other people have an aspirin allergy that triggers wheezing or growth of nasal polyps.

If you take too much aspirin, your ears may ring, your hearing may be muffled, or your vision may blur. (Oddly enough, if you're hard of hearing, you may not know your ears are ringing, making it hard to recognize this sign of overdose. The woman described in the *New England Journal of Medicine* was hard of hearing, which is probably why she thought the ringing was music.)

As for plain old aspirin, it's hardly plain anymore. In recent years, drug companies have introduced a wide array of aspirin products, available in new forms and containing a variety of nonaspirin ingredients. If your doctor recommends aspirin for your arthritis, use this guide to help you sort out what's available.

Plain aspirin. These pills contain *only* aspirin (acetylsalicylic acid) and perhaps some inactive ingredients such as potato starch, hydrogenated vegetable oil, or calcium phosphate to hold the pill together. If your stomach can tolerate it, plain aspirin is the cheapest arthritis medication there is, and it works fine. (For some tips on how to minimize stomach irritation, see the discussion of nonsteroidal anti-inflammatory drugs—a group to which aspirin belongs—later in this chapter.)

Coated aspirin. These aspirin tablets have a protective coating that allows them to pass through the stomach and dissolve in the small intestine, thus causing less upset and irritation than plain aspirin. Ecotrin, for example, has a coating that contains cellulose, a natural plant material. If you can't stomach plain aspirin, doctors say these tablets are worth a try. Sometimes, however, the coating keeps the aspirin from dissolving properly, preventing absorption.

Buffered aspirin. Some aspirin brands, such as Ascriptin and Bufferin, contain antacids. The idea is that the antacids will neutralize the secretion of excess stomach acid that is triggered by aspirin. But most doctors say that buffered aspirin is no better than plain aspirin. The amount of buffer added is too small to do any good, says Paul Plotz, M.D., an aspirin expert at the Arthritis and Rheumatism Branch of the National Institutes of Health. Buffered aspirin also costs more than plain aspirin. If your stomach bothers you, take aspirin with an over-the-counter liquid antacid such as Maalox (which has more buffering action than a tablet), or ask your doctor for a prescription antacid. (Food acts as an excellent buffer, so taking aspirin with meals is another option.)

Arthritis-strength aspirin. Aspirin brands such as Arthritis Pain Formula contain more aspirin per tablet, which means you can take fewer pills and get the same effect. A standard regular-strength aspirin tablet has 325 milligrams of the drug; one tablet of Arthritis Pain Formula has 500 milligrams. This type of aspirin may be a good choice if you find it inconvenient or difficult to swallow a lot of pills.

Timed-release aspirin. One form of aspirin, Zorprin (zero-order release), releases aspirin slowly and steadily into your system rather than dissolving quickly in your stomach like plain aspirin. The big advantage of this long-acting aspirin is that you usually need just two tablets twice a day. Zorprin, which requires a prescription, also causes less stomach upset than regular aspirin.

Trilisate (and other brands of choline magnesium trisalicylate). This drug is less irritating to the stomach than regular aspirin. Like aspirin, Trilisate is broken down by digestion to yield an active ingredient called salicylate. The difference between these two medicines is in the parent compounds they contain. The salicylate in aspirin comes from acetylsalicylic acid. The salicylate in Trilisate comes from a mixture of choline salicylate and magnesium salicylate. Two closely related formulas are Disalcid and Magan. These drugs also break down to yield salicylate but are less toxic than aspirin because they, too, come from different parent compounds. People who are allergic to aspirin often can take all these close relatives of aspirin safely. One major difference, however, is that they require a prescription and are more expensive.

There's no need to bother buying aspirin brands with extra ingredients, such as caffeine or acetaminophen. Acetaminophen (brand name Tylenol) is a pain reliever that doesn't fight inflammation. Beware, too, of taking aspirin along with other over-the-counter remedies such as Alka-Seltzer, Midol, and Sine-Off. These and other nonprescription products also contain aspirin, so you might unintentionally take an overdose. When in doubt, check the label. (For a quick reference guide to aspirin and other arthritis drugs, see "Common Arthritis Drugs and Their Side Effects" on page 228.)

Nonsteroidal
Anti-Inflammatory Drugs

Nonsteroidal anti-inflammatory drugs are commonly known as NSAIDs (pronounced "ensaids"). They work the same way as aspirin does to fight pain and inflammation and may produce similar side effects.

In some ways, these newcomers are an improvement over aspirin. They're more potent, so you can take fewer pills and achieve the same effect. (One of the NSAIDs, Feldene, can be taken just once a day.) On the other hand, they cost a lot more than aspirin. And almost all require a prescription. Generally, these drugs are easier on the stomach than plain, uncoated aspirin, although they still cause their share of problems, including occasional ulcers.

Although ibuprofen (a leading NSAID) is available without a prescription in the form of Advil, Nuprin, and other brands, most people with arthritis don't buy the drug over the counter. Instead, they usually take a higher-strength form of ibuprofen, such as Motrin or Rufen, that requires a prescription. (The prescription form allows you to take fewer pills and actually costs less per milligram than Advil at a dosage of, say, 2,400 to 3,200 milligrams per day.)

Some prescription-only NSAIDs cause worse problems than others. Indocin (chemical name indomethacin) can have unpleasant effects on the nervous system, causing headaches, dizziness, and depression. Worst of all is Butazolidin (chemical name phenylbutazone), which can cause a fatal form of anemia. "Phenylbutazone probably should be taken off the market," says Dr. Plotz. "I don't think it has any unique properties that make it especially valuable any more." Other doctors say Butazolidin has limited use in some cases of severe arthritis that can't be helped by milder medicines.

For the most part, doctors don't even pretend to be scientific about deciding which NSAIDs to prescribe. Despite how closely these drugs resemble aspirin—and each other—their effectiveness

(continued on page 220)

Test Your Drug IQ

Quick, what's the molecular formula for methotrexate?

Just kidding. You don't need a Ph.D. in chemistry to demystify drugs. But you do need a basic working knowledge of their proper use. Take this quiz to see how much practical information you know.

The Questions

1. Among the foods you might take with your medicine to reduce stomach upset, a glass of milk is the ideal choice. True _____ False _____

2. If your aspirin bottle smells like vinegar, it's time to replace it. True _____ False _____

3. If you forget to take a scheduled pill, you should simply take twice as much the next time. True _____ False _____

4. The best place to store your medicines is in the bathroom. True _____ False _____

5. It doesn't matter whether you lie down or stand up to take a pill. True _____ False _____

6. If you encounter unpleasant side effects from oral corticosteroids, you should call your doctor but not discontinue the drug abruptly. True _____ False _____

7. Even on days when you feel good, you should continue taking your arthritis medications, unless your doctor says otherwise. True _____ False _____

8. If your arthritis medicine doesn't work within a week, it's never going to do you any good. True _____ False _____

The Answers

1. False. Surprisingly, milk is not a good choice, because its abundant protein stimulates the release of stomach acid, possibly causing more

218

upset. Other foods that may irritate your stomach are tomato, orange, and grapefruit juices. A banana, an English muffin, and applesauce are better choices.

2. True. A vinegarlike odor means the aspirin is decomposing; throw it out.

3. False. By taking twice your normal dose, you risk toxic side effects or an overdose. It's wiser to call your doctor's office and ask how to get back on schedule. Better yet, next time you get a new prescription, ask beforehand what to do if you forget a pill.

4. False. The bathroom is too humid for safe storage of many medicines. Find a cool, dry, dark, childproof place instead, such as a locked desk drawer.

5. False. If you lie down, a pill can sit in your esophagus for a long time, delaying relief and increasing irritation. Stand or walk around for at least 15 minutes after taking pills so gravity can help get them down into your stomach faster. Also, always take your pills with water to flush them all the way down your throat. (Some antihypertensive medicines, taken to control high blood pressure, can make you dizzy. You may want to lie down if you feel such ill effects.)

6. True. These drugs need to be tapered off gradually, not stopped abruptly. Because they suppress the natural production of corticosteroids, your body needs time to start production again.

7. True. With many arthritis drugs, you need a steady blood level in your system day after day for best results. Changing the dose upsets this balance and may keep the drug from working effectively.

8. False. Some arthritis drugs take months to work. Even aspirin may need up to six weeks to achieve its full anti-inflammatory effect.

varies from person to person. "It's largely a matter of trial and error," says Dr. Lisse. He suggests that his patients keep a diary for several weeks, noting how well an NSAID works. To monitor effectiveness, jot down such things as how long morning stiffness lasts, how much pain occurs (on a scale of 1 to 10), and how easy it is to get dressed or do chores. (It may take two or three weeks for you to assess a drug's effects.) If a drug isn't satisfactory, it may be worth trying another NSAID for a few weeks. Some people have to experiment with several NSAIDs before they find the one that works for them.

Aspirin or any of the NSAIDs can irritate your stomach, so be on the alert for signs of an ulcer. Notify your doctor promptly if you have any of these symptoms.

- A stomachache that wakes you up at night.
- Stomach pain between meals that's relieved by food.
- Persistent loss of appetite or nausea.

Also see your doctor if you experience foot swelling, ringing in the ears, wheezing, or high fever.

Seek medical help immediately, even if you have to go to the emergency room, if you:

- Vomit blood.
- Pass reddish or dark, tarry stools. (This is a sign of blood loss from the intestine.)

To lessen the chance of stomach upset or ulcers, try taking aspirin or NSAIDs after meals or a snack. Or try the pill-sandwich method: Eat some food, take your pills, then eat some more food. Also, limit or avoid the use of alcohol, which adds to the corrosive effect of NSAIDs on your stomach. And talk with your doctor about using antacids.

Disease-Modifying Anti-Rheumatic Drugs

Doctors often try aspirin or an NSAID to relieve the symptoms of RA at first. But if these relatively mild and safe drugs don't work, they turn to more powerful (and potentially toxic) medicines, such as gold, penicillamine, antimalarial drugs or methotrexate, which are collectively called DMARDs, for disease-modifying anti-rheumatic drugs. Although these drugs work in different ways, all have the potential to dramatically reduce joint pain and swelling. In fact, they can result in remission—a total absence of any signs of the disease, and they're being used earlier in RA, to the point where most patients are being treated with them. To keep the disease in check, you generally have to keep taking the drug.

If you can't tolerate one kind of DMARD, your doctor may recommend you stop taking the drug and try another. Similarly, if you don't get a good response from one, you may have success with another. It's not unusual for people to try two or three DMARDs until they find one that best relieves their symptoms with no side effects—or minimal ones.

Here's a run-down of the DMARDs.

Gold therapy. Gold has been used to treat RA for more than 50 years, although no one knows exactly how it relieves joint pain and swelling. Most people receive gold in the form of weekly injections—it usually takes three to four months of shots before the treatment starts to work. About 60 percent of people who are treated with gold shots get excellent results, according to Arthritis Foundation estimates. Another 30 percent stop because of side effects, and the remaining 10 percent get no benefit at all.

Gold pills (brand name Ridaura) recently became available, and studies show that they are no less effective than injections. Nevertheless, many rheumatologists feel that the pills aren't quite as effective as the shots, despite their convenience. Also, gold pills cause diarrhea in 40 percent of the people who take them—far more than the number who suffer diarrhea from gold shots. And while the pills are less toxic than shots, you'll still have to be stuck with a needle every month or so for routine blood tests. (These tests are necessary to monitor for harmful side effects, including damage to the kidneys or bone marrow.)

Penicillamine. Sometimes people who aren't helped by gold do have a good response to penicillamine (brand names Depen and Cuprimine), a chemical cousin to the antibiotic penicillin. How penicillamine works is not understood. You'll have to wait several months to know whether or not the drug works for you. As for side effects, penicillamine can cause blood and kidney damage, so routine blood and urine tests are necessary. Rarely, this drug can trigger other autoimmune diseases, including lupus and myasthenia gravis (a neuromuscular disease).

Antimalarial drugs. It's not quite clear why antimalarial drugs such as hydroxychloroquine (brand name Plaquenil) can sometimes relieve RA. The antimalarials, however, are considered less effective than other slow-acting drugs. They also can cause irreversible damage to the retina. Although this side effect is rare, people on hydroxychloroquine must have frequent eye exams to detect drug-induced changes in the retina before vision is impaired. Otherwise, they're probably safer than gold or penicillamine, which is why they're tried first, says Dr. Lisse.

Methotrexate. People who don't benefit from gold or other slow-acting drugs sometimes do well on methotrexate. More commonly used as an anti-cancer drug, methotrexate is used in far smaller amounts to treat RA. Methotrexate relieves arthritis symptoms faster than gold or penicillamine, often bringing improvement in just a few weeks. About 60 percent of those who try it have less joint pain, swelling, and stiffness, sometimes remarkably so, says Michael Weinblatt, M.D., assistant professor of medicine at Harvard Medical School and director of the Robert B. Brigham Arthritis Center in Boston. People who take methotrexate must not drink alcohol, because the combination increases the risk of liver damage, hepatitis, and other liver disease.

"For me, methotrexate is like a miracle drug," says Simon Pomgratz, one of Dr. Weinblatt's patients. Until he began taking methotrexate five years ago, nothing helped Pomgratz's RA. "Methotrexate was the only drug that helped me. It not only helped me, it practically did away with my arthritis. I no longer have pain and swelling in my joints. It changed my life completely."

Generally, people try methotrexate only if they have not had a good response on gold or penicillamine. Although methotrexate works well for some people, it's no wonder drug. Because it works by suppressing the immune system, it has the potential to cause serious side effects, including damage to the bone marrow, liver, and lungs.

Closely related drugs reserved for difficult cases of RA are aza-thioprine (brand name Imuran), which some doctors say works more slowly than methotrexate, and cyclophosphamide (brand name Cytoxan), which is more powerful but also more toxic. These drugs (especially cyclophosphamide) carry a slight but definite risk of causing cancer or leukemia.

When should these powerful medicines be deployed? Many doctors are turning toward earlier treatment with these drugs in the hope of preventing joint damage. However, these drugs are used only after milder medicines, namely aspirin and other NSAIDs, have been tried and prove to be unsatisfactory for controlling arthritis. (Other, more experimental drugs are discussed in chapter 18, "Frontiers in Arthritis Research.")

Cortisone

When a new drug called cortisone was introduced shortly after World War II, people with severe arthritis jumped—or at least walked—for joy. Within days of taking the drug, bedridden patients could walk again without pain. The world marveled that the cure for arthritis had been found, and the Nobel Prize for Medicine was bestowed on the doctors who developed the drug.

If all this seemed too good to be true, it was. Within a few years, doctors and patients became aware of the many side effects of the cortisone family of drugs. These drugs, all closely related to a group of natural hormones called corticosteroids, can dramatically suppress pain and inflammation. But their long-term side effects, which include ulcers and suppression of the immune system, can be worse than the disease.

Howard MacDonald knows the side effects all too well. He took Decadron (one of the most powerful cortisonelike drugs) for many years. While the drug helped to ease his joint pain and swelling, it's also responsible for two cataracts, a "buffalo hump" on his upper back, weak muscles, thin skin, and osteoporosis.

"When steroids were first introduced, doctors used them freely to treat arthritis, and many people experienced harmful side effects," says Dr. Lisse. Today, doctors are far more prudent in their use of these drugs. When steroids are needed for long-term therapy, such as to treat lupus, serious RA, or a few other conditions, doctors try to use the smallest effective amounts to minimize side effects.

Sometimes corticosteroids are used for short-term therapy. Someone with RA, for example, might take very low doses of corticosteroids for two or three months until their gold shots begin to work. "Oral corticosteroids are never recommended for people with osteoarthritis," says Dr. Lisse.

A steroid shot can practically be a cure for some joint problems, such as shoulder bursitis or tennis elbow (a common form of tendinitis). By suppressing the inflammation, the steroid helps the joint to heal. But using steroids for bursitis or tennis elbow shouldn't be confused with using them for arthritis. And steroids should not be injected into a problem joint more than two or three times a year because repeated injections can damage the joint. (Don't confuse a steroid injection into an inflamed joint with an intramuscular shot in the arm or buttocks. A joint injection just relieves the problem joint, while an intramuscular shot is absorbed into the bloodstream and affects the whole body.)

Anti-Gout Drugs

If you have gout, you can still eat, drink, and be merry (in moderation, of course). Years ago, gout sufferers were told to avoid such foods as liver, sardines, fish roe, and sweetbreads, which can raise uric acid levels and trigger a gout attack. But thanks to modern medicine, now you can have your caviar and eat it, too. Doctors say watching your diet is not as effective a way to prevent gout attacks as medicine. "Gout is essentially a controllable disease now," says Bruce Hoffman, M.D., chief of rheumatology at the Medical College of Pennsylvania in Philadelphia.

For people with infrequent gout attacks, the only drug that's needed is an NSAID such as Clinoril, Naprosyn, or Indocin. Taken at the first twinge of pain, these drugs bring prompt pain relief and stop the flare-up. Another prescription drug, colchicine, also can shut down a gout attack altogether if taken early in the attack, although its potential side effects include nausea and diarrhea.

By the way, if you wake up at 3:00 A.M. and suspect your gout is flaring up, don't reach for aspirin: Doctors say it's the *last* thing you should consider for gout because in small doses, aspirin can raise blood uric acid levels—the very condition that got you into trouble with gout in the first place. Acetaminophen won't help much either, because it's not an anti-inflammatory drug. If you've been prescribed an NSAID or colchicine for gout, keep refills handy at home or when you travel.

If you have frequent gout attacks or are at risk for developing deposits of uric acid in your kidney or elsewhere, your doctor may prescribe long-term drugs to lower your blood uric acid levels. Two medicines, Probenecid and Sulfinpyrazone, clear the body of uric acid by increasing its excretion by the kidneys. Another drug, allopurinol, reduces production of uric acid. Colchicine also works to prevent gout attacks, although no one knows exactly why. In any case, all these drugs prevent uric acid from precipitating into the needlelike crystals that can inflame joints and cause kidney stones.

Don't take anti-gout drugs unless you're certain you have gout. That may sound like silly advice, but gout is commonly misdiagnosed, say Dr. Hoffman and many other rheumatologists. Although many people have high blood uric acid levels, only a small number of them suffer from gout attacks. The rest are perfectly healthy and don't need anti-gout drugs. Yet some doctors wrongly prescribe anti-gout drugs for everyone with high blood uric acid levels. Generally, rheumatologists don't recommend anti-gout drugs until someone suffers a first gout attack. The diagnosis also should be confirmed by checking a sample from the inflamed joint for the telltale uric acid crystals.

A Controversial Arthritis Drug

Thomas McPherson Brown, M.D., director of the Arthritis Institute at the National Orthopedic and Rehabilitation Hospital in Arlington, Virginia, believes RA is caused by a tiny infectious agent called a mycoplasma—and he claims he cures patients with the common antibiotic tetracycline. In the book *The Road Back,* Dr. Brown and coauthor Henry Scammell state that "tetracycline ther-

Twelve Tips for Safer Drug Use

No drug is perfectly safe or totally free of possible side effects. To minimize the disadvantages of taking medicine to relieve arthritis, follow these tips.

• Learn all you can about a new drug before you take it. Always read the package insert with a drug (prescription or nonprescription), and follow the instructions to the letter. If you have any questions, contact your doctor, nurse, or druggist.

• Ask your doctor about foods you should avoid while taking any of this medicine. Find out if alcohol or nicotine will interfere with the drug or enhance side effects. Ask if the new drug will affect any other medicines, including over-the-counter remedies, that you take for other health problems.

• Tell your doctor if you have any known or suspected allergies to any drugs.

• Before taking a new drug, ask your doctor what side effects are possible and what to do if adverse reactions occur. Find out if any side effects would require emergency care. Tell your doctor promptly if adverse reactions occur.

• If you are over 60, ask your doctor if you need to take any special precautions when taking medicine. The physical changes that accompany aging may affect the way your body reacts to drugs.

• Find out if it's okay to drive a car, work on a ladder, operate power tools, or perform other potentially hazardous activities while taking your medicine.

apy is the only effective therapy to reach toward the cure of rheumatoid arthritis"—to which some members of the medical establishment reply, "Balderdash."

"It's irrational," says Dr. Plotz. "Using tetracycline to treat rheumatoid arthritis is irrational, not supported by any scientific evidence. What's more, antibiotic drugs are not without side effects, and they probably are without benefit." While Dr. Plotz and other doctors are open-minded and recognize that infection may

- Don't take any drug in the dark. Make sure there's enough light so you can accurately identify the drug and take the proper dose. If you wear glasses, put them on to read the label before taking your medicine.
- Tell your doctor if you are pregnant while taking any medicine, prescription or nonprescription.
- Shake all liquid forms of drug to make sure the ingredients are mixed thoroughly before you swallow the medicine.
- Ask your pharmacist for a standard measuring spoon; a kitchen measuring spoon may not be accurate.
- If you have trouble opening bottles of pills, ask your druggist to repackage your medicine in easy-to-open containers instead of bottles with childproof caps. Or ask a friend to open them for you, then repackage the pills in more convenient dispensers. (Be sure to keep *all* medicines well out of the reach of children.)
- To help you keep track of your medications, consider carrying a pocket diary, where you can jot down the correct times to take scheduled doses throughout the day. Or, you can buy an inexpensive calendar-type dispenser for the drugs you take. These are small containers that store your prescription in compartments, one for each day of the week. Another suggestion: Buy an inexpensive alarm wristwatch, which can be easily set to beep at various times throughout the day to remind you to take your pills.

play some role in RA, they caution that no one has yet proven what causes it, let alone that tetracycline is *the* cure.

Still, what have you got to lose if you do try this treatment? It depends. If none of the conventional treatments have relieved you, then taking a long shot with tetracycline might be worth a try. Keep in mind, though, that tetracycline isn't entirely harmless. The drug sometimes causes diarrhea— which may be helped by eating yo-

(continued on page 236)

Common Arthritis Drugs and Their Side Effects

Generic Name (brand name)	Use	Possible Side Effects
Aspirin		
Aspirin (Bayer, Ecotrin, others)	In low doses, relieves pain and reduces fever. In higher doses, also acts as an anti-inflammatory drug to treat rheumatoid arthritis, osteoarthritis, and other musculoskeletal conditions.	Stomach irritation is most common problem, including heartburn, nausea, indigestion, and loss of appetite. Can lead to stomach bleeding or ulcers. (Stools will be black or tarry; see doctor at once.) In high doses, can cause hearing loss (especially in the elderly), ringing in ears, dizziness, and confusion. Rarely, causes damage to blood cell production, liver, or kidneys.
Nonsteroidal Anti-Inflammatory Drugs (NSAIDs)		
Ibuprofen (Motrin, Rufen)	Used to relieve symptoms of rheumatoid arthritis, osteoarthritis, bursitis, tendinitis, and related conditions.	Similar to those of aspirin. Common gastrointestinal problems include heartburn, nausea, indigestion, loss of appetite, and possibly, bleeding ulcers. May cause swelling from water retention (may raise blood pressure), dizziness, headache, or ringing in ears. Rarely causes hearing loss, blurred vision, kidney damage, or anemia. In elderly, prolonged use can cause confusion.
Indomethacin (Indocin, Indocin-SR)	Same as other NSAIDs.	Similar to those of other NSAIDs. In addition, may cause confusion or forgetfulness. Gastrointestinal side effects may be more severe than those for other drugs in this group.
Meclofenamate (Meclomen)	Same as other NSAIDs.	Similar to those of other NSAIDs, although diarrhea may be more common.
Naproxen (Naprosyn, Anaprox)	Same as other NSAIDs.	Similar to those of other NSAIDs.

	Precautions	**Interactions with Other Medications**
	Don't use if you are allergic to aspirin (symptoms are wheezing and nasal polyps) or NSAIDs. Don't use if you have stomach ulcers or a bleeding disorder such as hemophilia. Avoid or limit intake of alcohol, which can increase gastrointestinal side effects.	Taken with oral anticoagulants, aspirin can increase the risk of bleeding. With NSAIDs (below), aspirin can increase the harmful side effects. With oral anti-diabetic drugs (including insulin), can sharply decrease blood sugar levels. Large doses of vitamin C can increase aspirin's toxicity.
	Don't take if you have a known allergy to this drug or to aspirin, if you have stomach ulcers, or if you are pregnant or nursing. Consult your doctor if you have liver, kidney, or heart problems or high blood pressure. Ibuprofen should not be used by people with lupus. Avoid or limit alcohol intake, which increases chances of stomach ulcers and bleeding.	This drug can decrease the effects of certain diuretics (furosemide, Lasix) and beta-blocker drugs. May also increase the toxic effects of lithium. Avoid prolonged use with high doses of acetaminophen (Tylenol), which may cause kidney damage. Concurrent use with aspirin may increase gastrointestinal side effects and may actually decrease the effectiveness of both drugs.
	Same as for other NSAIDs.	Same as other NSAIDs.
	Same as for other NSAIDs.	Same as other NSAIDs.
	Same as for other NSAIDs.	Same as other NSAIDs.

(continued)

Common Arthritis Drugs and Their Side Effects
Continued

Generic Name (brand name)	Use	Possible Side Effects
Nonsteroidal Anti-Inflammatory Drugs (NSAIDS)—*Continued*		
Phenylbutazone (Butazolidin)	Short-term treatment of severe ankylosing spondylitis or other joint diseases that don't respond to milder drugs.	Harsher than those of other NSAIDs. Common problems are nausea, heartburn, indigestion, and occasional vomiting. Water retention may occur, possibly raising blood pressure or, rarely, causing congestive heart failure. Can cause a rare and fatal form of anemia.
Piroxicam (Feldene)	Same as other NSAIDs.	Similar to those of other NSAIDs.
Tolmetin (Tolectin; Tolectin DS)	Same as other NSAIDs.	Similar to those of other NSAIDs.
Sulindac (Clinoril)	Same as other NSAIDs.	Similar to those of other NSAIDs.
Disease-Modifying Drugs for Rheumatoid Arthritis		
Gold shots (Myochrysine, Solganal)	Slow-acting drug that can often suppress pain, swelling, and other symptoms of rheumatoid arthritis and may prevent later deformities.	Pain at injection site. Skin rashes, mouth ulcers, and metallic taste in mouth are common. Most serious potential problems are kidney damage or damage to bone marrow, suppressing blood cell production. More toxic than other oral drugs in this category.
Oral gold (Ridaura)	Same as gold shots.	Same as gold shots, plus 40 percent of patients have diarrhea.
Penicillamine (Cuprimine, Depen)	Same as gold.	Fever, chills, or rash may occur in first month. Less-serious side effects are mouth ulcers, loss of taste, and metallic taste in mouth. Rarely, can cause blood or kidney damage or trigger autoimmune disorders.

Precautions	Interactions with Other Medications
Use with great caution, under close supervision of a rheumatologist.	Same as other NSAIDs.
Same as for other NSAIDs.	Same as other NSAIDs.
Same as for other NSAIDs.	Same as other NSAIDs.
Same as for other NSAIDs.	Same as other NSAIDs.
Don't take if you are allergic to gold or other heavy metals, or if you have liver, kidney, heart, or blood disease or high blood pressure.	Should not be used with penicillamine. Side effects may be increased with concurrent use of other drugs that are toxic to liver, kidneys, or bone marrow.
Same as for gold shots.	Same as gold shots.
Don't take if you are allergic to this drug, have kidney problems, or are pregnant.	Should not be used with other drugs that might damage blood or kidneys, such as gold, antimalarials, methotrexate, or phenylbutazone.

(continued)

231

Common Arthritis Drugs and Their Side Effects
Continued

Generic Name (brand name)	Use	Possible Side Effects
Disease-Modifying Drugs for Rheumatoid Arthritis—*Continued*		
Hydroxy chloroquine (Plaquenil)	Same as gold, also used to treat lupus.	May cause skin rash, nausea, vomiting, diarrhea, muscle weakness, nervousness, headache, or dizziness. Rarely, causes damage to retina, but this can be monitored (and therefore prevented) with regular eye exams.
Methotrexate	Used in small doses to suppress the symptoms of rheumatoid arthritis and sometimes psoriatic arthritis. Works faster than other drugs in this group.	Most common are nausea, upset stomach, loss of appetite, and rarely, diarrhea and vomiting. Can cause liver or lung damage. Also, reversible depression of sperm count, causing male sterility. Rarely, suppresses bone marrow, causing anemia or too few white blood cells.
Azathioprine (Imuran)	Same as methotrexate, but sometimes takes longer to work.	Nausea, heartburn, and vomiting are most common problems. Can cause bone marrow suppression, leading to anemia or too few white blood cells. Slight but definite risk of cancer or leukemia, liver problems, or pancreatic inflammation.
Anti-Gout Drugs		
Allopurinol (Zyloprim)	Helps prevent gout by reducing uric acid production. Not useful for acute gout attack.	Most common are diarrhea, nausea, and drowsiness. Call doctor immediately if you have skin rash, painful urination, bloody urine, or swollen lips or mouth. Rarely, can damage blood cells, liver, or other internal organs.

| | Interactions with Other |
Precautions	Medications
Don't take if you are allergic to this drug or are pregnant or nursing. Consult your doctor if you suffer from alcoholism or liver disease. May exacerbate certain inherited blood disorders.	Should not be used with drugs known to damage the liver.
Don't take if you are deficient in folate, malnourished, have chronic liver or kidney disease, or are a heavy drinker. Don't take if you are pregnant or nursing. Use with caution if you have lung disease. Do not drink while taking methotrexate.	Never take with antibiotics Bactrim or Septra.
Not recommended if you are pregnant or nursing or have an infection.	Effect and toxicity can be increased by the anti-gout drug allopurinol (Zyloprim). May decrease effects of oral anticoagulants and certain muscle relaxants.
Use with caution if you have liver or kidney problems or if you're allergic to sulfa drugs.	Can increase toxic side effects of azathioprine. Taken with antibiotics like ampicillin, allopurinol increases risk of skin rash. Taken with oral anticoagulants, may increase risk of bleeding.

(continued)

Common Arthritis Drugs and Their Side Effects
Continued

Generic Name (brand name)	Use	Possible Side Effects
Anti-Gout Drugs—*Continued*		
Colchicine (Novocolchine)	Used both to prevent gout and relieve an acute attack.	Dose-related diarrhea, nausea, and stomach pain are signs to stop taking the drug and check with your doctor. Signs of severe overdose are bloody urine, stomach burning, severe vomiting, or seizures. Overdose can cause rare but fatal anemia. Rarely, causes damage to blood cells, kidney or other organs.
Probenecid (Benemid)	Helps to prevent gout by increasing the excretion of uric acid. Not useful for acute gout attack.	Side effects are uncommon, but can include headache, loss of appetite, nausea, or vomiting. Call doctor if you notice lower back pain, painful urination, or bloody urine. Rarely, causes damage to kidney, liver, or blood cells.
Oral Corticosteroids		
Prednisone, prednisolone, methyprednisolone (Medrol)	Used to suppress symptoms of rheumatoid arthritis, lupus, and certain other inflammatory diseases.	Side effects are more common if drugs are taken for a long time or in high doses. Can cause increased appetite, weight gain, a rounded "moon" face, hump on upper back, easy bruising, slow wound healing, increased risk of infection, stomach upset, increased growth of body hair, diabetes, cataracts, acne, muscle weakness, bone thinning, and emotional problems.

NOTE: This table does not list all drugs prescribed for arthritis, and it does not include all side effects, adverse reactions, or contraindications for each drug listed. For additional information, consult the package inserts provided with prescription drugs (available from your pharmacist), the current edition of *Physicians' Desk Reference* (carried by many libraries), or your physician.

Precautions	Interactions with Other Medications
Don't use if you are allergic to this drug. Check with doctor if you have blood disorders or kidney, liver, or heart disease.	Can decrease the effect of anticoagulants and increase the effect of some mood-altering drugs (narcotics, sedatives, tranquilizers). Can increase the toxicity of phenylbutazone.
Don't use if you are allergic to this drug. Check with doctor if you have a kidney, liver, or blood disorder.	Can increase the effects of oral anti-diabetic drugs. Should not be used with aspirin. Can increase the toxicity of penicillin and methotrexate.
If drug is used for long-term therapy, don't discontinue abruptly.	Sodium-containing medications may cause swelling and increased blood pressure. While on corticosteroids, immunization with live virus vaccines is not recommended.

gurt but can also be life-threatening—or vaginitis. Infrequently, it causes skin rash, hives, itching, stomach upset, or irritation of the mouth. There's also a small chance that by disrupting the body's natural milieu of microorganisms, the drug may invite the growth of new and more harmful germs. So if you haven't tried the standard arthritis drugs, such as aspirin or gold, you're not doing yourself any favors by considering tetracycline. By giving up an opportunity to try a proven medicine, you might suffer joint damage that otherwise could have been prevented. Tetracycline therapy can take many months to work, according to Dr. Brown. But if it doesn't work, you've lost valuable time. So be careful.

Arthritis Drugs and Your Diet

A number of common arthritis drugs interfere with the body's use of minerals and vitamins. With some drugs, you may need more of a particular nutrient than usual. If so, try to get these extra nutrients from foods rather than a supplement, advises Glen Thompson, Pharm.D., a clinical pharmacist at the University of Alabama who has studied the effect of arthritis drugs on nutrition. The following list will help you determine if arthritis drugs are interfering with your diet.

Aspirin. If you take a lot of aspirin, make sure you get enough folate, an essential B vitamin. Aspirin can lower the body's folate level, and a deficiency can cause anemia. Good sources of folate are liver, wheat germ, dark, leafy green vegetables, and legumes. Aspirin also can increase vitamin C excretion, so eat your share of citrus fruits, strawberries, green peppers, and tomatoes. Don't take vitamin C supplements, however; they may increase aspirin's toxicity.

NSAIDs. If you take aspirin or any other NSAIDs, you may be losing blood from your stomach, small intestine, or esophagus. Iron lost with this blood must be replaced so your body can make new red blood cells. To replace iron, eat liver, meat, leafy green vegetables, dried apricots, raisins, nuts, and whole grains.

Oral corticosteroids. These drugs alter mineral metabolism in several ways. First, by increasing sodium and water retention, steroids can cause water weight gain (most often noticeable as swollen ankles) and increase blood pressure. To counteract these effects, avoid sodium-rich foods, such as salty snacks, canned soups, and pickled or cured foods. Second, steroids speed up the loss of two other minerals: zinc and potassium. Oysters, liver, nuts, cheese, eggs, grains, and poultry are high in zinc. Meat, potatoes, melons, and bananas are rich in potassium.

Corticosteroids also tend to break down protein in the body and can cause muscle wasting, activate latent diabetes, or increase insulin requirements in diabetics.

Aluminum- or magnesium-containing antacids. These medicines, if used regularly, interfere with phosphorus absorption. If that happens, the body responds by withdrawing both phosphate and calcium from bones. The result may be thinner, more fragile bones, also known as osteoporosis. Low-fat dairy products are good sources of phosphorus and calcium.

Penicillamine. This drug can inactivate vitamin B_6, so some doctors recommend supplements of the B vitamin when the drug is prescribed. Tingling in your hands and feet is a sign of B_6 deficiency. Wheat germ, meat, liver, whole grains, peanuts, and corn are rich in B_6. Supplements above the Recommended Dietary Allowance (2.2 milligrams for men, 2.0 milligrams for women) shouldn't be taken without a doctor's approval and supervision.

Methotrexate. This drug should not be used by people who are deficient in folate, says Dr. Weinblatt. A deficiency of this B vitamin may magnify the drug's harmful side effects, he says. Liver, yeast, green leafy vegetables, and legumes are rich sources of this nutrient.

Taking folate supplements may negate the drug's side effects, says Dr. Lisse.

CHAPTER

15

Who's Who on Your Health Care Team

Score: Arthritis, 50, Linda Hoover, 0. That's how lopsided and dismal Linda's situation looked when she first got rheumatoid arthritis (RA). She didn't even know what she was fighting, and she already felt beaten by pain, stress, and fatigue.

But Hoover, an upbeat and outgoing mother of two, was no quitter. Instead, she enlisted the help of a winning team of arthritis health professionals, including a rheumatologist, a nurse, an occupational therapist, a physical therapist, and a social worker. In short, she teamed up with folks who play hardball against arthritis—and won.

Hoover's doctor worked on choosing the best medicines. Her nurse alerted her to possible side effects. Her occupational therapist showed her how to cope with stress and fitted her for a beautiful silver ring that doubles as a miniature splint to rest and support a particularly achy finger. Her physical therapist designed a home exercise program that made her feel good and strong again. And her social worker became a kind and supportive friend, always ready to listen. Together and separately, these professionals at St. Margaret Memorial Hospital in Pittsburgh rallied to support Linda. They helped her to beat arthritis. These days, Hoover looks and feels like the winner she is.

"My physician is a wonderful person, but he's only one person and can't do everything," she says. "All these people are very highly trained in their individual areas. They complement each other. They show you what you can do and how well you can do it." Together they make arthritis management a positive, whole-body program, she says.

If you have arthritis, don't be a bench warmer. Sign on with a team of arthritis health professionals and get on with the game. In many communities, you can find most or all of these experts working together under one roof in arthritis clinics or hospitals. But even if your doctor works in a small practice, he can still refer you to other helping professionals. This chapter will give you an idea of what kind of help these pros have to offer. Although you might not need the services of all of them, you're likely to benefit from one or two who can coach you—and help you score big points against arthritis.

Is a Specialist Always Necessary?

If you have arthritis, going to see a doctor is an important decision. But even more crucial is seeing the right doctor, because the wrong treatment—or a misdiagnosis—can be as bad as no treatment at all.

Consider the experience of Kathleen Kennedy, a Philadelphia woman who visited five doctors over 15 years before finally learning why her arms ached so much. Shortly after her first child was born, Kennedy, then 29, found her arms so sore she could hardly pick up her baby. "I constantly ached, ached, ached," she says. The first doctor she consulted, a family physician, couldn't find anything wrong. "This doctor looked at me as though he thought, 'What a hypochondriac!' " says Kennedy. "He said he didn't know what the problem was." Her next three doctors, all orthopedic surgeons, did treat her knees for unrelated osteoarthritis. But none had a clue why her arms continued to hurt, so she continued to suffer in frustration.

Finally, at age 44, Kennedy's luck improved. A relative suggested she see a rheumatologist, a doctor who specializes in arthritis. At last she got a diagnosis: She had fibromyalgia (also called fibrositis), a common condition that causes pain without other obvious physical signs like swelling and redness. "I thought, 'Well, thank the Lord. I'm not a crackpot after all!'" she says with a good-natured laugh. "I was elated that I had a recognizable—and treatable—problem. So in a way, going to see a rheumatologist was the best thing that ever happened to me. He knew what to look for."

In many cases, a family doctor may be the only physician you'll need to see for your arthritis. Should you feel you need someone with more expertise, however, consider going to a rheumatologist. These doctors are specialists in internal medicine (and occasionally pediatrics) who have an additional two to three years' training in arthritis and joint diseases. They're qualified to treat the more than 100 kinds of arthritis.

If you're undecided about whether you should see a rheumatologist, ask yourself these questions.

1. Is my doctor unable to diagnose my problem, despite several office visits or laboratory tests?

2. Am I getting little or no relief from my present treatment?

3. Has my doctor diagnosed arthritis but insists that nothing can be done, that "You'll just have to learn to live with it?"

4. Have I been diagnosed as having RA, lupus, or any other serious form of arthritis?

5. Have I been diagnosed as having a rare type of arthritis such as scleroderma, ankylosing spondylitis, or polymyositis?

6. Has my doctor failed to refer me to other arthritis health professionals, such as a physical therapist or an occupational therapist who may be able to help?

7. Has my doctor suggested treating my arthritis with gold, methotrexate, penicillamine, or other powerful but risky drugs?

"If you answered yes to any of those questions, a visit to a rheumatologist may be wise. Even if you know what your problem is, a rheumatologist can confirm the diagnosis and reassure you about its treatment," says Bruce Hoffman, M.D., chief of rheumatology at the Medical College of Pennsylvania in Philadelphia. (Relatively easy-to-manage bursitis, tendinitis, or osteoarthritis may not require a second opinion, however.)

One way to find a rheumatologist is simply to ask your family doctor for a referral. Or call your local chapter of the Arthritis Foundation for a list of specialists in your area. Also, ask friends and neighbors who have arthritis if they can recommend any rheumatologists. If you do consult with a rheumatologist, you still have several options about your future care. You can opt to continue being treated primarily by your family doctor, who can consult with the rheumatologist from time to time if necessary. Or you may decide to switch to the rheumatologist for all your arthritis care.

Other Bone and Joint Doctors to Consider

Rheumatologists are not the only doctors who know joints inside out.

Orthopedic surgeons.   Also called orthopedists, many orthopedic surgeons treat people with arthritis. After finishing medical school, these doctors spend one year in general surgery, then receive four years of surgical training on joints, bones, and the rest of the musculoskeletal system. Their skills include installing artificial joints, removing diseased joint linings, and realigning bones to relieve joint pain. (These remedies are discussed in chapter 17, "Are You a Candidate for Surgery?")

If you have a relatively simple case of bursitis, tendinitis, or osteoarthritis, you'll get basically the same care from an orthopedist or a rheumatologist. But in general, rheumatologists are better able to handle more complex types of arthritis, such as gout, ankylosing spondylitis, fibromyalgia, lupus, or RA. (If you don't know what you have, see a rheumatologist.)

Physiatrists.   During the course of your treatment, you may also be referred to a physiatrist (pronounced fiz-ee-AT-rist), a medical doctor who specializes in treating people with physical disabilities of various types. A physiatrist can orchestrate your physical therapy, most likely prescribing exercises, biofeedback, the use of heat and cold, and other physical treatments. If you have severe arthritis and need a lot of rehabilitation, a physiatrist can make a *big* difference.

Podiatrists. If your feet or ankles bother you, a podiatrist may be of special help. These doctors spend four years learning foot medicine in podiatric medical school, then complete a one- to three-year residency program in a hospital. Not surprisingly, proper footwear is the mainstay of podiatric medicine.

"To an arthritis patient, footwear is as therapeutic as steroids or any other medication," says Charles L. Jones, D.P.M., vice president of academic affairs and dean at the Dr. William M. Scholl College of Podiatric Medicine in Chicago. Podatrists'often prescribe special shoes or shoe inserts called orthotics to help arthritis. By keeping your feet correctly aligned and supported, the right shoes can reduce stress on your feet and other weight-bearing joints, possibly relieving pain from your toes to your back.

Podiatrists may also prescribe drugs or perform surgery to correct arthritis problems in the feet and ankles. However, if your foot symptoms are part of a bigger problem, such as gout or RA, the podiatrist will usually work with a rheumatologist.

Physical Therapy for Pain Relief and Mobility

Shortly after Kathleen Kennedy learned she had fibromyalgia, her doctor suggested she see a physical therapist. At first, she was skeptical. After all, her complaint was pain, not lack of mobility. "I thought, why physical therapy? What is physical therapy going to do? I'll go, but this is really a waste of time."

But Kennedy soon learned that physical therapists do much more than limber up stiff joints with therapeutic exercises. Although they are not medical doctors, these licensed health professionals are skilled in pain management and can show you how to use heat or cold treatments to soothe aching joints. They also use sophisticated devices to reduce chronic pain, such as TENS (transcutaneous electrical nerve stimulation), a painless form of electrotherapy, or therapeutic ultrasound.

In Kennedy's case, a physical therapist taught her some relaxation exercises (including a variation of Progressive Relaxation) and suggested some tapes to listen to. The treatment proved better at preventing pain than any medicine she has tried. "The physical therapist told me she was going to teach me to relax. And I said, 'Honey, if you can do that, it'll be a miracle.' And guess what? She did it! She gave me the tools to relax. And she showed me that I am in charge of this thing."

If you have trouble walking or moving any joints, a physical therapist may be able to show you the best range-of-motion, stretching, or isometric exercises for your particular condition. Often the therapist will serve as your teacher, giving you a set of exercises to do at home. If you want to start an aerobic exercise program, a physical therapist can tell you how to work out safely. And if you need a cane, wheelchair, or walker, this professional can help you select the right one and use it correctly.

"Anybody who has a diagnosis of arthritis should see a physical therapist at least once," says Jodi Maron-Barth, a physical therapist who works with arthritis patients at Moss Rehabilitation Hospital in Philadelphia. "In one visit alone, you can be educated for a lifetime."

In most states, you'll need a referral from a doctor to see a physical therapist. If your doctor can't recommend one who works with arthritis patients, call your local chapter of the Arthritis Foundation. Or write to the American Physical Therapy Association, 1111 North Fairfax Street, Alexandria, VA 22314.

When to See an Occupational Therapist

What's your line? Are you a career person, a parent, a homemaker, a community volunteer—or all of the above? No matter what roles you juggle in life, an occupational therapist can show you how to get your jobs done with a minimum of pain, stress, and fatigue.

Don't assume that occupational therapists help only those who work at jobs in offices and factories. Homebodies benefit, too. These licensed health professionals can show you how to rearrange your kitchen to make cooking and cleanup easier. They can tell you about self-help aids that make getting dressed or taking a shower a snap. And they can work with you and your employer to figure out how to make your job manageable despite arthritis.

But an occupational therapist's role goes far beyond showing you how to use a button aid or a long-handled toothbrush. "The occupational therapist gets you thinking about how the disease is affecting your life and how to rearrange your schedule and activities to make the best of it," says Cynthia Stabenow Kulp, a registered occupational therapist and an instructor who works with arthritis patients at the University of Virginia Medical Center in Charlottesville. "And the occupational therapist may be the one to help you accept the fact that perhaps you can't do everything you could before you got arthritis."

Linda Hoover, for example, sat down with her occupational therapist and made a list of what she does—or tries to do—in a typical day. Then she ranked the importance of each activity. Taking care of her two small children was her top priority. But at the same time she realized that a lot of routine household chores caused her pain and fatigue, leaving her tired and cross by dinnertime. As a result, her kids got shortchanged. So instead of trying to keep the family's three-story Tudor home spic-and-span, she decided to hire a cleaning person. She also set limits on her volunteer activities. As a result, Hoover has the energy she needs to take care of her family.

An occupational therapist can teach you how to protect your joints from unnecessary stress when performing everyday tasks like opening a jar of pickles or planting tomatoes in your garden. A therapist can also fashion a wrist or hand splint to wear when your joints need a rest and teach you how to cope with stress. As with physical therapists, you'll need a referral from your doctor to see an occupational therapist. If your doctor can't recommend one, call your local chapter of the Arthritis Foundation or check with the rehabilitation department of any large hospital.

An Arthritis Nurse Specialist: A New Breed of Caregiver

A newly emerging specialty is evolving among nurses: the arthritis nurse specialist who, through experience more than formal training, can fill the various helping roles of teacher, comforting friend, nutritional adviser, exercise consultant, and arthritis drug expert. You might say your nurse is a Jack (or Jill) of many medical trades.

"The nurse seems to be the individual who crosses over into a lot of different areas," says JoAnn Weaver, R.N., rheumatology coordinator of the Arthritis Center of Nebraska in Lincoln. "An arthritis clinic may not have a physical therapist or a registered pharmacist, but it almost always has a nurse."

Nurses see their primary job as teaching you what you need to know about arthritis to live independently. They can advise you about taking your medicines, getting enough rest, and doing your exercises correctly. They also have lots of special tips for people with arthritis. If you're taking drugs that reduce your appetite or interfere with good nutrition, for example, a nurse may be able to offer dietary advice. Nurses also know how to comfort people in pain and can show you how to relax or sleep more comfortably. At many clinics, nurses give patients medicines that have been prescribed, such as weekly gold shots. (In addition to being R.N.'s and L.P.N.'s, some nurses are certified nurse practitioners.)

Perhaps most important, a nurse is often one who finds time to listen and offer advice. "Many times, the patient may be reluctant to ask the doctor certain things. They're afraid they'll take up too much of the doctor's time," says Weaver. "A nurse may be easier to talk to."

Where to Go for Emotional Support

Sometimes arthritis deals the deepest blow, not to your body but to your spirit. "Often people with arthritis become depressed because they can no longer do what they used to do, and they see themselves as being less of a person," says Stephen Wegener, Ph.D., a clinical psychologist who counsels arthritis patients at the University of Virginia Health Sciences Center in Charlottesville. "A psychologist can help the person rebuild his or her self-esteem."

Banishing the blues is just one way a psychologist can improve your outlook. Besides helping to heal the emotional pain that arthritis can inflict, a psychologist can offer practical guidance. Here are some of the major reasons to consider seeing a psychologist.

• Do you have chronic pain that's not relieved by drugs, exercise, and other physical treatments? A psychologist may help you to relieve pain naturally, by teaching you self-hypnosis or other relaxation methods, or how to distract your attention from pain with pleasant imagery or other techniques.

• Does arthritis keep you awake at night? Sleep problems are more common among people with arthritis, says Dr. Wegener. By showing you how to improve your sleep habits and relax before bedtime, a psychologist may help you snooze soundly again.

• Is arthritis putting a damper on your love life? If pain is disrupting an intimate relationship, a psychologist may help you and your partner work together toward a solution.

• Do you have trouble following your doctor's advice? A psychologist can help you set up a plan to reward yourself for sticking to an exercise program or other treatments. This professional also can help you accept the fact that you have arthritis and encourage you to get on with your life.

To find a psychologist, ask a rheumatologist if he knows of one who works with arthritis patients. If not (these specialists are somewhat rare), look for a psychologist with experience in managing chronic pain or helping people with other disabilities. If your community has a pain clinic, there may be a psychologist on staff who can help. Look for a licensed psychologist with a Ph.D. in counseling or clinical psychology. Or your doctor may suggest a psychiatrist, a medical doctor who diagnoses and treats mental or emotional problems. If so, look for a psychiatrist who specializes in managing pain or coping with chronic diseases.

The Social Worker: More Than Sympathy

Ever feel like sticking your head out the window and screaming, "I'm not going to take it anymore!" Tell it to your social worker, who is there to listen and be supportive.

Like psychologists, social workers are trained as counselors. They can help you deal with feelings of anger, depression, and guilt that often come with being sick. Besides supporting those who have arthritis, a social worker can talk to other family members, who may be confused or upset or may not understand the changes taking place. "We work on getting the family involved," says Rodney L. Rutkowski, a medical social worker who works with arthritis patients at St. Margaret Memorial Hospital. "If a person has the support of the people around them, they don't feel isolated, and they can respond much better. Sometimes, they just need to hear someone say, 'I love you,' or 'I care about you.' "

Even if your family and friends are real troupers, you may feel like a candidate for primal scream therapy because you're getting the runaround from government agencies that are supposed to help. In that case, a medical social worker may be able to make short work of red tape. These professionals know what kind of financial help and community resources are available to you, from Meals-on-Wheels or similar programs run by the National Association of Meal Programs to Social Security Disability Insurance.

If you're hospitalized for arthritis, a medical social worker may act as the "discharge planner"—the person who makes arrangements for any follow-up care you need at home. In an arthritis clinic, a social worker also can serve as a patient advocate, acting as a go-between between you and your doctor if you're not satisfied with your progress or have questions about your treatment. Many of these skilled caregivers also can teach you how to cope with stress.

If a social worker might be of some help to you, ask your doctor for a referral to a medical social worker who has a master's, or M.S.W., degree. Your local chapter of the Arthritis Foundation also may know of medical social workers in your area. Or you can call the social work department of a local hospital.

When to Turn to a Dietitian

"For years, I've told doctors that I cannot eat citrus fruit, tomatoes, strawberries, or any fruit except bananas without suffering joint pain for two or three days," complains Samuel Pugh, an Indianapolis man who has RA. "But all they say is, 'Diet has nothing to do with arthritis.' "

As Pugh and many others have learned, getting sound nutritional advice about arthritis is not easy. And no wonder. Out of almost 2,000 members in the Arthritis Health Professions Association, only six were listed as dietitians or nutritionists in 1987. Yet a dietitian or qualified nutritionist may help if your doctor has advised you to lose weight or if your medication calls for a special diet (for example, a low-salt diet for corticosteroids).

So if you do need dietary advice, don't give up your quest for help, for there are qualified experts who can work with you. "If you suspect some kind of sensitivity or allergy to food, there are lots of dietitians who can help," says Patricia H. Harper, a registered dietitian who is a nutritional consultant in Pittsburgh. "You probably aren't going to find a dietitian who specializes in arthritis, but you will find dietitians who are very knowledgeable about food allergies."

To find a dietitian, ask your doctor for a referral or contact your local hospital's dietitian. You might also consult a nutritionist, but look for someone with a Ph.D. in nutrition science from a reputable college or university.

Your Pharmacist Can Help, Too

Are you wondering whether it's okay to have a drink or two while taking your new medication? If an over-the-counter allergy remedy will interfere with your arthritis pills? For everything you ever wanted to know about drugs but were afraid to ask your busy doctor, turn to your pharmacist.

Your neighborhood pharmacist can probably answer almost any drug-related question you may have. After all, pharmacists spend three years studying drugs in pharmacy school, giving them a broader education on the subject than most doctors.

In many drugstores, a pharmacist can store your medical history in a computer, so when you come in to have a new prescription filled, he can search through data on thousands of possible drug interactions in a flash, making sure the prescription won't interfere with your other medications. Ideally, your doctor should check for the same problems, but the task can be monumental, and the pharmacist can serve as a valuable safety check. Pharmacists may also be able to compare the costs of different medications and recommend generic equivalents.

You may also find a helpful pharmacist at a large arthritis clinic or hospital. At Spain Rehabilitation Center in Birmingham, Alabama, for example, clinical pharmacist Diann Peoples educates people with arthritis about their medicines and works with doctors to select the best drugs for each patient. "Studies have shown that the more people know about their medicines, the more compliant they are," she says.

And taking the right medicine at the right time in the right way helps bring the relief that the drugs are intended to produce.

16

Alternative Remedies:
Proceed with Caution

Somewhere in the Southwest, an elderly woman called her local chapter of the Arthritis Foundation with an unusual inquiry. "I understand that standing naked under an almond tree in the full moon cures arthritis," she said. "Do you have an enclosed area with an almond tree where I can go for this treatment?"

Every year in Montana, thousands of people with arthritis flock to old uranium mines, hoping to soak up the supposed curative powers of radioactive gas.

In Pennsylvania, a farmer claims to have cured his sister's severe arthritis with manure. "I simply buried the limbs of my sister in warm cow manure, covering with an oilcloth to retain heat, and changed the packs three times a day," he reported.

Still other people have been snookered by an arthritis remedy that sounds out of this world: moon dust. Unfortunately, the alleged moon dust was ordinary sand from planet Earth. The cost of this rip-off: $100 for 3 ounces.

Quack remedies: Some are harmless, some are dangerous, some are disgusting—and all are useless. Sometimes, bogus remedies are even amusing—until you stop to think how many innocent and vulnerable people are victimized by them and how much money they spend.

Nine out of every ten people with arthritis try an unproven remedy (that is, a treatment that scientists have not shown to be safe and effective), says Wilbur Blechman, M.D., a rheumatologist and former chairman of the Arthritis Foundation's Subcommittee on Unproven Remedies. In addition to visits to uranium mines and other practices mentioned earlier, these alleged (but unproven) "miracle cures" include (but aren't limited to) mud, colonic irrigations, water, light, and even voodoo!

These worthless pills, potions, and gadgets aren't cheap, either. People with arthritis spend more than $2 billion a year on quack treatments, according to a congressional subcommittee that investigated quackery. To put that into perspective: For every $25 that was spent on bogus treatments in one recent year, only $1 was spent on legitimate scientific research for arthritis.

Health Fraud Kills

Unfortunately, hucksters can rob you of your health as well as your life savings. "Unproven remedies do more than take money from gullible people," states Floyd C. Pennington, Ph.D., the Arthritis Foundation's spokesman for unproven remedies. "The use of dangerous, unproven remedies kills far more people than we'll ever know." While most alternative treatments are relatively safe, some are dangerous. Some people have become very ill after receiving hazardous arthritis drugs in Mexican border clinics. And it appears that one woman died from a snake-venom injection she received for arthritis. Even a seemingly harmless folk remedy, such as wearing a copper bracelet, can hurt you if you delay seeking proper medical care.

It's not hard to understand why people seek alternative treatments, though. "When you have years of pain and anguish, you will try anything, within the bounds of safety," writes Christiaan Barnard, M.D., in his book, *Christiaan Barnard's Program for Living with Arthritis.* Dr. Barnard speaks from experience. The world-famous heart surgeon suffers from rheumatoid arthritis (RA) and has tried numerous unproven treatments. "I make no bones about admitting to sampling homemade pure honey, ginseng root, and even royal jelly [made by bees]," he writes.

Not all nontraditional healers push worthless treatments, though. Some offer reasonable options, particularly for arthritis sufferers who feel dissatisfied or frustrated with conventional medical care. Chiropractors, for example, sometimes are more successful than traditional doctors in treating bad backs and other common arthritis ailments. And clinical ecologists, who make up a controversial medical specialty that emerged a few years ago, have claimed a fair amount of success treating people who have a kind of arthritis linked to food or chemical allergies.

How to Size Up "Miracle" Cures

How do you, the medical care consumer, tell a legitimate and knowledgeable alternative healer from a self-serving promoter of bogus remedies? To help you distinguish between alternative therapies that are safe (and possibly worthwhile) and those that are harmless (or downright dangerous) and useless, Dr. Pennington and other experts offer these guidelines.

Investigate the remedy before trying it. Ask lots of questions—how it works and what side effects it can trigger, for example—just as you would if you were considering a new prescription drug or having surgery. Have studies proven it effective? (You may want to ask to see copies of the studies.) What medical credentials and experience does the practitioner have? How much will it cost? Most important, what possible harm might result from the therapy? Reliable sources of information include the Arthritis Foundation, your doctor, or self-help books like this one. And by all means, write to the company and demand evidence to support claims. If you aren't satisfied with what you find, pass.

Don't give up your regular medical care to try an alternative remedy. Unconventional healers do not have the same training and experience in diagnosing or treating arthritis as rheumatologists and other traditional health professionals. Should you choose an alternative healing method, consider it as an addition to, rather than a substitute for, your regular care. If you plan to substitute an alternative therapy for traditional care, consider asking your doctor to monitor your progress with regular checkups.

Tell your doctor about any unproven remedies you try. Your physician needs to know if an alternative treatment will interfere with your medications or other therapies. Some herbal remedies, for example, contain active ingredients that may block or counteract the effect of your medications. Your doctor also may have more information to share about an alternative treatment.

Take a cautious, "try-it-and-see" approach. A little skepticism is healthy. Before you make a big commitment to an unproven therapy, decide how much time and money you're willing to spend to see results. That way, if the treatment doesn't work, your loss will be minimal. "Don't worry about offending your physician by questioning his judgment," says Jeffrey Lisse, M.D., assistant professor of rheumatology at the University of Texas Medical Branch, Galveston, Texas. "He (or she) is doing you a service."

Watch out for hucksters and zealots who claim their treatment is the one-and-only answer to your problem. Most people with arthritis benefit from a combination of therapies, not a single type of treatment. (For tips on spotting a health hoax of any kind, see "How to Duck a Quack" on page 254.)

Clinical Ecology and "Allergic Arthritis"

If you suspect your arthritis is aggravated by certain foods, you might seek help from a clinical ecologist. Also called doctors of environmental medicine, these specialists are physicians with either an M.D. or D.O. (doctor of osteopathy) degree. They believe that food allergies frequently trigger the symptoms of RA and other forms of arthritis (among other diseases). They also believe that common chemicals in our homes and workplaces can cause some forms of arthritis. If so, the most effective and common treatment is to avoid whatever triggers your symptoms—and the list of suspected causes can be long. Clinical ecologists use arthritis drugs only as a last resort.

It's hardly likely that your hips or knees could waste away to practically nothing because you ate or breathed something that doesn't agree with you. But clinical ecologists believe substances in

How to Duck a Quack

Does a product advertised as an arthritis remedy seem too good to be true? Put it to the test. The following tips, gleaned from the Arthritis Foundation and the Better Business Bureau, will help you avoid a health hoax and suggest what to do if you have fallen prey to a medical quack.

Watch out for arthritis remedies sold by high-pressure salespeople. One-time deals or treatments that require you to pay a lot of money up front also are clues that something is wrong.

Beware of remedies that promise instant relief or a miraculous cure. The more dramatic and sensational a claim sounds, the less likely it is to be true. "Miraculous water from Lourdes heals thousands!" is a typical example.

Be leery of advertisements that use testimonials from allegedly satisfied users. A typical statement is "The miracle water is wonderful. We are so much better. I wouldn't want to do without it!" from someone you can't contact, such as "Mrs. A. R., Florence, KY." Testimonials are not a substitute for scientific studies of a product's safety and effectiveness.

Be cautious of practitioners who encourage you to avoid legitimate health care providers. Hucksters often try to drum up support for their products by fostering distrust of traditional medicine. They may accuse doctors of prescribing needless surgery or dangerous drugs, while contending that their own product is the only safe and effective treatment.

the environment can cause various kinds of arthritis flare-ups. Some people with RA, for example, have an allergic reaction to certain foods, which causes their joints to become hot and swollen—much like pollen makes hay fever sufferers sneeze. Other cases of arthritis may result from sensitivity to man-made chemicals, says William J. Rea, M.D., a prominent clinical ecologist and director of the Environmental Health Center of Dallas. Sensitivity to chemicals may cause arthritis through a different mechanism than food allergy, he adds, although no one is sure what that mechanism is.

Don't use remedies that come without directions, a list of ingredients, or warnings about possible side effects. Unlabeled products can contain harmful chemicals or ingredients that may interfere with other medications you're taking.

Be leery of products that tout all-natural ingredients. Just because something is natural doesn't mean it's harmless. Cobra venom is natural, for example, but it's hardly a safe arthritis remedy.

Watch out for ads that claim a product is endorsed by state or federal agencies, such as the Food and Drug Administration. These agencies are not allowed to issue endorsements, so such claims are probably false.

If you feel you have been victimized by a quack, there are several steps you can take to help yourself and others. Here's what to do.

Stop using the remedy or gadget. If the product has harmed you, contact your physician. Your doctor may ask you to bring the product to his or her office, along with any information you have about it.

Report the problem to the appropriate government agencies. This may protect others from an unsafe remedy. Offices to contact include your local chapter of the Arthritis Foundation, the Better Business Bureau, the Attorney General's office, the Food and Drug Administration, and the U.S. Postal Service (for mail-order fraud).

Clinical ecologists say allergic reactions and chemical sensitivities are important causes of RA and lupus and may also play a role in fibromyalgia and osteoarthritis. But so far, only a few scientific studies have been done to try to confirm these hunches. Rheumatologists counter that there's no good evidence for such claims.

Yet clinical ecology seems to help some people with arthritis. "It worked for me," says Charles Voors, 67. Voors had severe RA that wasn't relieved by aspirin and other standard drugs. His rheumatologists predicted he would end up in a wheelchair. So Voors sought help from a well-known clinical ecologist, who found that his arthritis was triggered by household sources of common chemicals (like gas or heating oil) and by foods treated with pesticides. Voors's treatment consisted of changing his diet and lifestyle to avoid the offending substances. He eats mostly organically grown foods to avoid pesticides and agricultural chemicals. He also moved into a new condominium with electric heat because fossil fuels caused his arthritis to flare up. Voors says these steps have almost completely relieved his arthritis, except for some lingering joint damage in his fingers and feet. Without this treatment, he says, "I would have ended up in a nursing home."

As gratifying as stories like this may sound, clinical ecology has some limitations. Because these doctors are not arthritis specialists, they may know little about splints, self-help devices, physical therapy, and other treatments proven to be of help for serious joint problems. They also have less skill than rheumatologists at diagnosing the various kinds of arthritis. You should know, too, that clinical ecology is a fairly new discipline, not well-known or accepted by the medical mainstream. Most rheumatologists feel that clinical ecologists overemphasize the role of allergy in triggering arthritis. "Clinical ecology testing is expensive," says Dr. Lisse, "and by avoiding things one at a time on your own, you may accomplish the same results more cheaply."

If you want to consult a clinical ecologist, you can receive a directory with names of physicians in your general area by sending $3 and a self-addressed, stamped, business-size envelope to the American Academy of Environmental Medicine, P.O. Box 16106, Denver, CO 80216.

What Chiropractors Have to Offer

If you're looking for a drug-free and hands-on treatment approach for arthritis, chiropractic medicine is an alternative to consider.

Chiropractors emphasize the importance of the spine to overall health and well-being. They believe that when the vertebrae are not in the proper position, the spinal nerves that pass through these bones are pinched, contributing to disorders elsewhere in the body. Chiropractors manipulate the spine to put any misaligned vertebrae, or "subluxations," back into place, thus helping to relieve pain.

Many chiropractors say that about half of their practice is arthritis-related. According to chiropractors interviewed for this book, most use spinal manipulation to treat arthritis. They may also massage and manipulate other affected joints, helping to restore mobility. Other treatments for arthritis used by chiropractors and M.D.'s include physical therapy, heat and cold treatments, acupuncture, TENS (a pain-control technique), and nutritional counseling.

If you visit a chiropractor, don't expect to hop right onto the massage table, however. The initial office visit usually begins with a detailed medical history, then a physical exam and a set of X rays, says Linda Bocchichio, D.C., a Long Island chiropractor. Chiropractors rely on X rays to help them evaluate the condition of the person's skeletal system.

Chiropractors are not licensed to prescribe drugs or perform surgery. For that reason, if you have a more serious form of arthritis, such as severe RA, lupus, or scleroderma, the chiropractor should refer you to a rheumatologist. (One important caution: The Arthritis Foundation's Dr. Blechman warns that chiropractic manipulation is not recommended for people who have osteoporosis because their bones are too fragile.)

For some people with arthritis, chiropractic care works as well as or better than traditional medicine. "We offer a conservative approach," says William Hogan, D.C., director of clinical sciences at the National College of Chiropractic in Lombard, Illinois. "Why have somebody take steroids and other drugs for arthritis when they can get just as effective a treatment with a more conservative approach?"

Word of mouth from people who go to chiropractors is one way to find a chiropractic doctor, or you can call your local or state chiropractic association, listed in your telephone directory. If you live near a chiropractic college, the clinic there will have especially up-to-date care, says Dr. Hogan.

Metal Jewelry
and Other Folk Remedies

Whenever a stubborn health problem affects millions but can't be cured, folk remedies spring up. Here are a few to watch out for.

Copper Bracelets

As folk remedies go, copper bracelets are relatively harmless. "The worst that can happen is your wrist will turn green," says Dr. Blechman. He adds, however, that people shouldn't put off visiting a doctor while waiting for a copper bracelet to work.

One researcher showed that people who wore copper bracelets absorbed tiny amounts of copper through their skin, too little to cause the body any harm. And despite the fact that people say they feel better while wearing a copper bracelet, doctors say there is no known medical reason for the bracelets to help arthritis. Doctors attribute this improvement to a placebo effect—you feel better simply because you expect to. (The placebo effect explains why many unproven remedies seem to work, say doctors.)

Alfalfa: Good for Cows, Lousy for Arthritis

Here's an arthritis remedy that does double duty as livestock feed. It's alfalfa, the cloverlike plant that's widely used as a cattle forage crop.

Alfalfa has been used for yĕars as a folk remedy for arthritis. Some people drink tea made from alfalfa seeds, while others swallow alfalfa tablets. A few years ago, a Texan promoted the healing powers of Honey Al-Fa Tea, a concoction of honey and alfalfa. This particular swill was said to cure arthritis, hay fever, muscle cramps, and other ailments. "Best of all, you will be able to produce healthy bouncing babies who will be whiz kids by the time they reach school age!" proclaim ads for the product.

The truth is, hot alfalfa tea is mostly hot air in terms of health benefits. No form of alfalfa has any known therapeutic benefit for arthritis. Drinking alfalfa-seed tea is probably harmless, although one doctor noted it can cause skin problems. All in all, you're better off leaving alfalfa to the likes of Bessie the Cow.

WD-40: The Squeaky Joint Gets the Grease

How's this for an industrial-strength solution for arthritis? It's WD-40, a commercial lubricant best known for its ability to fight corrosion and keep machine parts working smoothly. (WD-40 can also be used to perform odd jobs around the house, such as freeing up "frozen" locks, for instance.)

The inexpensive lubricant is advertised as being able to "stop squeaks, loosen rusted parts, and free sticky mechanisms." So some folks have concluded that WD-40 can free up their own rusty hinges! Users spray it on stiff, achy joints. Apparently, WD-40 was first used as a painkiller by some farmers, who accidentally got the lubricant on their arthritic joints while spraying farm machinery. The farmers contended they got relief, and news of the folk remedy spread faster than, well; oil on water. The WD-40 Company, based in San Diego, makes no health claims for its product, yet it receives at least one letter a week from people who claim the spray lubricant gives them temporary relief from arthritis, says Louis Repaci, the manager of marketing services.

"We know of no reason why WD-40 should be effective in treatment of arthritis, and we do not recommend it for medicinal purposes," says Repaci. The Arthritis Foundation agrees whole-heartedly.

The WD-40 Company knows of no harm from getting WD-40 on the skin, although some people may develop an allergic rash from the product, which contains petroleum distillates. (WD-40 may be harmful or fatal if swallowed, and inhaling any aerosol has unknown but possibly harmful effects.) Needless to say, this is one arthritis remedy people can do without.

Stay Out of Radioactive "Health" Mines

Can people with arthritis find relief down in the pits? Thousands of desperate people who flock year-round to old uranium mines near Boulder, Montana, think so. They believe that the radioactive radon gas in the mines has curative powers for every form of arthritis. (That's right, radon—the same invisible but deadly gas that most people try to *avoid*.)

Visitors come from all over the world, many on crutches or in wheelchairs, to visit mines with such names as Merry Widow, Earth Angel, and Free Enterprise. They pay from $2.50 to $4 an hour to sit on benches located deep in the mine tunnels, breathing the radon gas that seeps from buried uranium ore and dipping their hands and feet in radioactive water.

Not only do medical experts dismiss radon therapy as bogus, they warn that repeated exposure to the radioactive gas can cause lung cancer. But mine visitors pay little heed. Stricken with lupus, RA, and other painful, often incurable conditions, they come in search of a medical miracle, seemingly oblivious to the potential dangers posed by this alleged "cure."

Jill Barta, 28, travels 1,000 miles from her Wisconsin home to visit the Free Enterprise Mine every year. She says that breathing the odorless and invisible radon gas is the only treatment that has helped her severe RA. "I've tried aloe vera, DMSO, alfalfa pills, gold shots, and aspirin. The mine is the only thing that works. If I didn't come here, I could be in a wheelchair in a short time."

While the benefits of radon gas are unproven, the dangers are well established. The National Academy of Sciences estimates that round-the-clock exposure to radon gas in homes causes 13,000 lung cancer deaths a year. And radiation levels in Free Enterprise Mine are several hundred times higher than the recommended upper limit of radon safety in homes.

Nevertheless, Montana state officials insist that mine visitors are at negligible risk for developing lung cancer. Despite the fact that visitors are allowed to stay in the mines for short periods only, no level of radioactivity is absolutely safe, says William Belanger, a radiation expert with the Environmental Protection Agency. "I certainly wouldn't do it," he says of visiting the mines. In fact, few if any experts can justify this controversial practice.

DMSO: Horse Liniment for People?

Is it a miraculous arthritis drug or just a great antifreeze? That's the riddle of DMSO, a common industrial solvent that's also a popular home remedy for arthritis. Proponents claim that rubbing DMSO into the skin improves circulation, relieves pain, and reduces swelling in achy muscles and joints. To hear some people talk, DMSO does everything but shine your shoes!

DMSO, which stands for dimethyl sulfoxide, is a by-product of the wood pulp manufacturing process. It is widely used in industry and as a veterinary medicine to treat horses and other animals. More than 20 million Americans also have tried DMSO to relieve sports injuries and arthritis. Most use DMSO as an ointment, rubbing it into the skin over a sprained ankle, tennis elbow, or other painful muscle or joint.

While proponents call DMSO a wonder drug, few doctors do. "I'm not impressed with it," says Raymond Adelizzi, D.O., chief of rheumatology and associate professor of medicine at the University of Medicine and Dentistry of New Jersey School of Osteopathic Medicine. A few years ago, Dr. Adelizzi tried to test the effects of DMSO as an ointment for arthritis in a double-blind study. But he had to abandon the trial halfway through. "We had too many patients who developed side effects, and roughly 90 percent of the side effects were due to the DMSO," he says.

Dr. Adelizzi says the most common adverse reactions to DMSO are skin rashes and itching, usually in the area where the drug is applied. Serious side effects are rare, but eye damage has been reported in laboratory animals. Occasionally, users also inject DMSO into the bloodstream, which can cause internal bleeding.

Even if you don't inject DMSO, it enters the bloodstream through the skin. Within minutes after it's applied, you'll smell like a head of garlic. ("That's putting it mildly," quips one doctor. "The fact is, if you sit down in a movie theater after applying DMSO to your skin, you'll trigger an exodus of patrons for five rows around you.") And when DMSO travels to the bloodstream, it carries with it anything that has made contact with the skin. Thus, if you rubbed DMSO onto your sore hands after gardening, you might end up with weed killer or fertilizer in your blood.

In the last 20 years, researchers have done hundreds of studies to test DMSO as a human medicine. Most doctors have concluded that although DMSO can temporarily relieve pain, it does not help the swelling and inflammation of severe arthritis. As a result, the Food and Drug Administration (FDA) has never approved DMSO for use as an arthritis drug. As a prescription drug, it is available only to treat interstitial cystitis, a rare and painful bladder disorder.

Where do people with arthritis get DMSO, if not from their doctors? Unfortunately, many people buy DMSO of questionable purity and strength at roadside stands, by mail order, or in paint and hardware stores. (The sale of DMSO is legal in ten states.) Solutions intended for industrial use can be dangerous because they contain harmful contaminants that get carried into the bloodstream by the DMSO. Why risk it?

The South-of-the-Border Rip-Off

Probably the most dangerous scams perpetrated against arthritis sufferers are the Mexican border clinics. These clinics, located near the California, Arizona, and Texas borders, lure Americans by promising to give them DMSO. The clinics are deceptive about the contents of the pills they dispense, however. Analysis of the pills has shown that what they really give unsuspecting patients is cortisone (among other substances), not DMSO. After taking cortisone, people return home feeling dramatically better. But in time, they may develop serious side effects, including bone thinning, muscle wasting, and cataracts. Sometimes the pills also contain tranquilizers and phenylbutazone, a drug that can cause fatal anemia. "It's true these people may feel better for a while," says Dr. Blechman. "But later they may develop severe side effects, and nobody is going to know why." Smart consumers will stick to legitimate U.S. medical centers.

Forget Bee Sting Therapy

It's hard to imagine a more cruel and painful treatment for arthritis than multiple bee stings. Yet, bee sting therapy has been around as an arthritis folk remedy for more than a century, and people continue to willfully seek out this exotic treatment today.

In Vermont, 83-year-old beekeeper Charles Mraz stays busy treating arthritis sufferers from all over the country with bee stings.

"I've been working with bee venom therapy for 53 years," he says proudly. "I've personally treated several thousand people."

Ready to shudder? Here's how it works: First Mraz feels the person's joints to find the most tender spots. Then he picks up a honeybee with a pair of tweezers, crushes it slightly, and presses the stinging end against a sensitive spot on the joint. This treatment is typically repeated until the joint is stung five or ten times. The person usually gets this treatment every other day until he or she is "cured."

Although ice is used to numb the skin before and after the ordeal, the stings still hurt like heck, says Mraz. Paradoxically, he believes the pain and swelling caused by the bee stings are necessary to make the treatment work—presumably by triggering a number of complex changes in the immune system. He claims bee sting therapy works to relieve all kinds of arthritis, including his own rheumatic fever years ago.

Most doctors, however, say bee sting therapy is for the birds. For one thing, bee stings can be deadly to people who are allergic to the venom. Allergic individuals may experience extreme swelling around the sting, develop hives, start wheezing, and possibly die. "Whether or not anyone has been seriously harmed, I don't know, but the potential certainly exists," says Dr. Blechman.

Scientists who have investigated this folk remedy say that someday purified components of bee venom might be used as legitimate arthritis medicines, perhaps in the form of an injection. Research on honeybee venom extracts has revealed several active ingredients that help to relieve experimental arthritis in animals. One ingredient triggers the body to release corticosteroids, naturally produced hormones that relieve pain and inflammation. Still, there's no good reason to endure the agony of bee sting therapy. When appropriate, doctors can prescribe these same hormones—painlessly—in pill form.

Snake Venom: Too Deadly to Consider

Snake venom is another potentially deadly arthritis remedy. A few years ago, people with arthritis began lining up at a Florida clinic, where a physician was giving injections made of cobra, water moccasin, and krait venoms. The mixture was said to cure both RA and multiple sclerosis. The doctor had teamed up with the owner of a local serpentarium, and the two men began shipping the venom to patients nationwide. A young Texas woman died while being treated, presumably because of a fatal reaction to the venom. The FDA finally stopped interstate sales of the venom, and the clinic went out of business. The use of snake venom for arthritis has never been scientifically investigated.

More Outlandish Arthritis Remedies That Got the Ax

If you thought using moon dust and cow manure were bizarre ways to relieve arthritis, you haven't heard anything yet. These phony cures were among those investigated—and condemned—by a congressional subcommittee on quackery.

The spectrochrome. Since everything else seems to cure arthritis, so must light. At least that was the dim-witted notion behind the spectrochrome, a big metal box with a 1,000-watt light bulb in it. The spectrochrome came with colored filters, used to change the color of the light. Red light was supposed to cure arthritis. But the treatment worked only if the patient stood nude and facing north when the moon was full! The FDA took this device off the market in the 1950s because—surprise—light does not cure arthritis. Occasionally, however, one surfaces, often in the hands of a practitioner who touts its alleged powers.

The vivicosmic disk. This gadget was a round disk, about the size of a silver dollar, which looked like a pumice stone. According to the promoters, dropping the disk into a glass of water gave the water special powers: It (allegedly) cured arthritis pain, and it also made a great deodorant and flu remedy! Needless to say, water of any kind has never been proved to cure arthritis.

Miracle Mud. For $9.95 plus $1 postage, the makers of Miracle Mud sent you 12 ounces of messy goo. Customers were told to "apply evenly over the affected joint and, if possible, cover with plastic food wrap. Within minutes, the soothing, deep-heating action will be felt." Deep heating is an understatement. Miracle Mud contained mustard and methyl salicylate, two blistering agents that can cause severe burns, especially if used with plastic wrap. Fortunately, the U.S. Postal Service stopped the sale of Miracle Mud.

The Kongo Kit. The kit consisted of two mittens and a belt, all made of hemp. The idea was that if you rubbed these items on the skin over an arthritic joint, the pain would go away. What really happened was that people inflicted so much pain on themselves by scouring their skin that they forgot about their arthritis.

The Sonus Film-O-Sonic. This gizmo was the brainchild of a California chiropractor, who promised to cure arthritis with music. The machine transmitted songs through electrodes attached to the skin. Arthritis was supposed to be relieved by songs like "Holiday on Strings."

Leg cramp leather bands. This device promised to relieve arthritis, along with leg cramps and muscle pulls. All you had to do was to slip the bands—actually, strips of leather or rubber—under your sheets at night. After reviewing this loony device, one physician remarked, "The only arthritis which can be improved or cured by this gadget is that in the lame brain of the promoter. No more need be said."

CHAPTER
17

Are You a Candidate for Surgery?

At best, joint surgery can bring dramatic pain relief, greatly improve your ability to use a joint, and allow you to return to a more active lifestyle. Just ask Betty Warner, 71, a veteran of arthritis surgery. Warner, who has severe rheumatoid arthritis (RA), says joint surgery saved her from living the rest of her life in a wheelchair. She has had seven joint operations, including surgery to replace both knees and hips with artificial joints. Thanks to surgery, she can walk a mile every morning, stay active with volunteer work, and socialize with her many friends. "I decided my disease was repairable, so I went out and got myself repaired," she says cheerfully.

Like Warner, more than 200,000 Americans a year undergo surgery to receive artificial joints, mostly new hips and knees. Most of these people tell dramatic stories about how this surgery has changed their lives for the better. For many, total joint replacement surgery has been the only salvation from excruciating, round-the-clock pain. And surgery restores their independence and dignity as well. Before surgery, many were so disabled they could not put on their own socks, comb their hair, or walk to the bathroom without a walker or cane for support.

The cause of such suffering: joints ravaged by arthritis. Severe osteoarthritis may completely wear away the cartilage in a knee, for example. Bill Warren, who received an artificial knee, remembers all too well how it felt to have no cartilage in his knee. "I had reached a point where if I stood for more than 10 minutes, the pain was so intense that I had to sit down. And if no chairs were available, I sat on the floor," he recalls.

While hip and knee replacements are the best-known forms of arthritis surgery, a number of other operations also are beneficial for certain kinds of arthritis. These options range from relatively minor procedures, such as shaving smooth the frayed cartilage in an arthritic knee, to other major procedures such as joint fusion, where the ends of the bones are fused together. Joints that have only mild to moderate damage, for example, often can be fixed with arthroscopic surgery. This revolutionary technique is a form of microsurgery that can be used to do many different operations. Arthroscopic surgery involves very little cutting of the tissues around the joint, so recovery is speedy and postoperative pain is minimal compared to some other, more extensive surgical procedures.

But surgery is serious business—certainly not a panacea for arthritis. Surgery can be painful and expensive and involve a long recovery period, keeping you away from work and limiting most other activities. With any operation, there also is the risk of serious complications. And if surgery is unsuccessful, the joint may be worse than it was before. So your best bet, before considering surgery, is to find out all you can about this option.

Arthroscopy for Diagnosis and Repair

You've heard of 1-hour dry cleaning, 30-minute pizza delivery, and express mail delivery. Well, now there's cut-and-go surgery. With a mini-operative technique called arthroscopic surgery, you can have your knee operated on in the afternoon and still be home in plenty of time for dinner.

Arthroscopic surgery is performed with miniature surgical tools inserted into a joint through quarter-inch incisions. Using an arthroscope (a pencil-thin telescope with a light on the end to illuminate the inside of the joint), the surgeon can examine the joint tissues for signs of disease. Or the image can be magnified, video-taped, and projected onto a television screen via a miniature camera on the arthroscope. A second tube, inserted through another incision, pumps in sterile fluid to expand the space in the joint, enabling the surgeon to manipulate his or her tools within the joint more easily and to wash out tissue debris.

Because the surgeon can actually see the tissue, arthroscopy can be used to diagnose complicated joint problems that elude X rays and other tests. Surgeons also can operate on joints by inserting tiny scalpels, drills, and other surgical tools through a third or fourth small incision. With arthroscopic surgery, surgeons can do most of the same operations that once required open joint surgery. Although most commonly used in the knee, arthroscopic surgery is being rapidly adapted for other joints, including the shoulder, ankle, wrist, elbow, hip, and jaw.

Arthroscopic surgery can be used to treat arthritis in various ways. For people with osteoarthritis, for example, the surgeon can remove painful bony spurs called osteophytes that grow around arthritic joints. Rough spots of cartilage can be shaved smooth, reducing pain and improving mobility. The surgeon also can suck out broken-off pieces of worn cartilage; these so-called loose bodies are painful and may cause a joint to lock. For those with RA, arthroscopic surgery is often used to remove diseased joint lining, helping to reduce pain and inflammation. (This procedure, called a synovectomy, is discussed in more detail later in the chapter.)

Many rheumatologists would not operate on someone with early arthritis in the knee—they would recommend conservative approaches, including physical therapy, exercise, or drugs, and save surgery for later, if necessary. "Arthroscopic surgery is not a first-line procedure," says Jeffrey Lisse, M.D., assistant professor of rheumatology at the University of Texas Medical Branch in Galveston.

Arthroscopic surgery is best suited to repairing mild to moderate joint damage. It is not a substitute for major operations, however. To repair severe joint damage, open surgical procedures, such as total joint replacement or joint fusion, are usually necessary.

"With arthroscopy, we can do basically all the operations that in the past would have required cutting the knee apart through 7-

to 10-inch incisions," says James M. Fox, M.D., medical director of the Center for Disorders of the Knee in Van Nuys, California, and staff member at the Southern California Sports Medicine Orthopedic Group. "What we've done with arthroscopy is caused the least amount of injury by surgery. We don't cut through major muscles or ligaments. We've saved the patient major disability from the surgery."

Most arthroscopic patients are admitted as outpatients in surgical clinics. The procedure is performed in an operating room, usually with general anesthesia. Generally, patients go home a few hours after surgery, using crutches for support if they've had knee arthroscopy. Usually, they need nothing more than a compressive bandage over their incisions.

The recovery time following arthroscopic surgery is half that following open joint surgery because there is less pain and immobilization after the operation, says Dr. Fox. A good example is a procedure called a meniscectomy, in which damaged or diseased cartilage between the bones in the knee is removed. With arthroscopic surgery, the patient goes home a few hours after the operation, requires crutches for only two or three days, and regains full range of motion within one to three weeks. With open joint surgery, in contrast, the same operation involves three to five days in the hospital, three to four weeks on crutches, and several months to regain full joint motion.

Know the Risks

Arthroscopic surgery is not risk-free, though. Although complications are less frequent than with open joint surgery, patients can develop blood clots or joint infections or have adverse reactions to anesthesia. Rarely, part of a surgical tool breaks off inside the joint, and if the surgeon can't retrieve it with arthroscopic tools, he may have to cut the joint open. In a few cases, people have lost limbs as a result of arthroscopic surgery because a major blood vessel was accidentally cut.

Sue Weston knows the possible consequences of arthroscopic surgery all too well. She had the surgery to remove smashed knee cartilage, caused by a hiking accident. Afterward, she was sent home on crutches without any warning about possible complications. A few days later, she woke up in agony, with the first of many postsurgical complications. Her leg felt as if it were on fire; it turned out her knee was bleeding internally, requiring emergency treatment. Not long after, she developed a serious infection in the knee, which put her in the hospital for five days. When that ordeal passed, she developed a blood clot in her lower leg, landing her back in the hospital for another ten days! Now, she says ruefully, "the joint is more damaged than it was to begin with." (Although Weston's ordeal began with an injury, not arthritis, the complications she encountered could happen to anyone undergoing arthroscopic surgery, regardless of why it was performed.)

Fortunately, horror stories like this are rare. Nevertheless, some surgeons are concerned that arthroscopy is being overused, exposing patients to needless risks. People whose joint problems are caused by sports injuries or accidents are more likely to have a questionable need for arthroscopic surgery than people who have RA, but everyone should consider all the consequences before consenting to this surgery, says Dr. Fox. "The lay public considers arthroscopy 'Band-Aid surgery,' and only a wimp or a four-year-old is afraid of a Band-Aid, so many people are absolutely fearless when it comes to arthroscopy," states Dr. Fox in his book, *Save Your Knees*. "I'm actually left in the bizarre position of having to talk some patients out of arthroscopic surgery. They tell me they have to have surgery because a friend of a friend had the exact same problem and is now running the Boston Marathon—backward."

If you're considering arthroscopic surgery for arthritis, here are some guidelines for using this technique wisely.

• Find a surgeon who is highly skilled in this delicate procedure. It may take several hundred operations for a surgeon to master arthroscopy. Also, an inexperienced surgeon may tend to exaggerate the degree of surgery needed because video magnification of the joint can make tissue damage appear more extensive or more serious than it really is.

• Find out if your doctor intends to use arthroscopy to diagnose a joint problem or repair it, or both. If the operation is solely for diagnosis, ask your surgeon if there are less invasive tests that could be used instead. Some forms of arthritis in the knee, for example, can be diagnosed with arthrography, a nonsurgical procedure in which a series of X rays is taken after dye is injected into the knee capsule. Many noninvasive diagnostic procedures are available; ask your doctor if any are appropriate.

• If arthroscopy is recommended to repair an arthritic joint, find out if there are other, more conservative options you could try first. Someone with an osteoarthritic knee, for example, might want to try physical therapy and drugs such as nonsteroidal anti-inflammatories (NSAIDs) to relieve pain before resorting to arthroscopic surgery. Or losing weight may relieve joint pain and postpone—or eliminate—the need for surgery. (See chapter 14, "What You Should Know about Arthritis Drugs" for more information about NSAIDs.)

• If you have arthroscopic surgery, don't rush back into action too soon, no matter how great you feel. "Although the incisions are small, people need to be reminded that they have had an operative procedure within the joint," says Dr. Fox. "Experience has shown that internal healing takes several weeks and, in fact, complete healing may take many months."

Joint Replacement Surgery: The Bionic Pain Reliever

How do you spell relief? If you have crippling arthritis that can't be helped by drugs and other conservative treatments, the answer may be total joint replacement (TJR). Essentially, the surgeon removes a badly damaged joint—most often a knee or hip—and replaces it with an artificial one made of metal and plastic. (You might say that the implant is an internal prosthesis for a hip gone bad.)

Amazingly, there are more than 200 models of artificial joints for the hip alone, although 10 models account for most operations. Surgeons also can custom-craft an artificial joint to fit an extra small or extra large person. In the hip, the prosthesis consists of two pieces: a plastic socket that replaces part of the pelvic bone and a metal component that replaces the worn-out part of the thigh bone. The metal component looks like a gearshift, with a long stem topped by a smooth ball. The stem fits inside the thigh bone, while the ball forms the new head of the thigh. The metal ball glides smoothly against the plastic socket, restoring easy motion.

In brief, here's how a hip replacement operation is done, as described by Earl C. Marmar, M.D., director of the Einstein-Moss Joint Replacement Center and assistant clinical professor of orthopedic surgery at Temple University School of Medicine in Philadelphia.

After the patient is anesthetized, the hip is exposed with a long incision and dislocated (that is to say, it's removed from the socket). The surgeon cuts off the top of the thigh bone, then cuts away diseased tissue in the hip socket and replaces it with the cup-like plastic socket. Then the surgeon hollows out a canal within the thigh bone and fills it with soft cement. Next, the long stem of the metal component is carefully eased down into the canal and pushed into place. In a few minutes, the cement dries around the stem, anchoring the implant securely.

Once these components are in place, the surgeon checks the hip's motion and stability, then closes the incision. This internal hardware fits so snugly that no cast is needed. The entire operation usually takes 2 to 3 hours. (Besides the chief surgeon, the surgical team may include two or three assisting surgeons, an anesthesiologist, and a scrub nurse.)

After such elaborate cutting and gluing, you might think you'd feel as though you'd been hit by a Mack truck. Surprisingly, many people have less pain immediately after the operation than they had just before it, says Dr. Marmar, because their arthritic hips are no longer there to torment them. "When I woke up from the anesthesia, I had no pain," marvels Howard MacDonald, who had his right hip replaced. Before his surgery, Howard felt round-the-clock pain from his badly damaged arthritic hip. Pain is an individual experience, however, and some people do feel discomfort after joint replacement surgery. Surgical pain usually goes away within two or three days, and it can be eased with medication. The hip operation also leaves an 8- to 12-inch scar, which some people occasionally find uncomfortable, says Dr. Marmar.

In general, though, TJR brings quick and dramatic pain relief. Bill Warren says his artificial knee ended 35 years of excruciating pain from osteoarthritis. "I'm now pain-free without any medication," he says. "It's as if the good Lord said, 'Bill, you've had all the pain you need.' And bingo, it was gone."

And freedom from pain is the primary reason people opt for new joints. Most people who receive artificial joints have advanced RA or osteoarthritis, often with excruciating pain from bone rubbing on bone, with nothing left to cushion the effects. Hip and knee replacements are the most successful—close to 95 percent of all patients report complete pain relief after surgery. Artificial implants also can relieve pain and restore function with a fair success rate in the shoulders, and to a lesser extent, in the ankles, wrists, and elbows. Artificial joints made of silicone are available for finger and toe joints.

Still, an artificial joint is no match for a healthy human joint. "If we do a good operation, the person may get back on the golf course and enjoy their golden years, but a hip replacement is not going to make them an Olympic athlete," says Richard Rothman, M.D., Ph.D., professor and chairman of orthopedic surgery at Thomas Jefferson University and chairman of the Rothman Orthopedic Institute at Pennsylvania Hospital in Philadelphia. The same is true in the knee and other joints. "I'm sorry to say bionic knees aren't going to have you leaping tall buildings in a single bound or even outpacing a lethargic dog named Bullet," says Dr. Fox.

Nevertheless, most people who have this surgery are thrilled with the results. MacDonald, who has completely recovered from his hip replacement surgery, says "It's just been a super, super thing. Now I can walk and do all the other things I should be able to do." Most recently, he traveled from his home in Philadelphia to England for a reunion with his World War II air force buddies. The trip would have been impossible before his surgery, he says. And a woman for whom just walking from her front door to her car was a torturous trek before surgery was able to dance at her son's wedding afterward.

What Can Go Wrong?

Like anyone who has TJR surgery, these folks faced a number of serious risks, and they knew it. A small number of people die from the surgery, usually because of a fatal blood clot in the lung.

At the Hospital for Special Surgery in New York, a highly regarded medical center that does about 1,500 joint replacements annually, about one to two people die of this complication each year, says Thomas P. Sculco, M.D., associate director of orthopedic surgery at the hospital and associate professor of orthopedics at Cornell University Medical College in New York City.

But the biggest problem with artificial joints is that they tend to fail over time. The metal and plastic can wear out (although they usually don't), and over the years, the cement that anchors an artificial joint to bone can crumble. When that happens, the implant wiggles out of its mooring, and pain and disability return. The longer you have an artificial joint, the greater the likelihood that the prosthesis will loosen from bone. With an artificial hip, for example, there's approximately a 10 percent chance the implant will loosen within ten years.

Unfortunately, if an artificial joint does loosen, the whole thing has to be surgically removed and replaced with a new prosthesis. This "revision" operation is more taxing than the original operation because the surgeon must spend time removing the original prosthesis and there is less bone on which to anchor the new implant.

Surgeons are excited about a new surgical advance that may reduce the problem of implants loosening. A "cementless" procedure has been developed that does not use glue to anchor the implant. Instead, the artificial joint is held in place by overgrowth of the person's own bone cells. So far, cementless operations are done primarily to replace hips. Although this form of TJR is still experimental, surgeons are hopeful these implants will last longer than cemented ones.

After a cementless hip operation, a person must use crutches for several weeks to keep most of his weight off the new joint. During this time, the bone is growing around the implant, and if too much stress is put on the artificial joint, it won't anchor itself securely in place. (The situation is different after a cemented hip operation. Since the cement dries so quickly, the hip is firmly anchored in place by the time the anesthetic wears off.)

People with artificial joints also must be on guard against infection for the rest of their lives. Artificial joints are not equipped to fight germs the way your own biological bones, tendons, and ligaments are, so they can become infected at any time by bacteria traveling from elsewhere in the body, like the bladder or an ingrown toenail. If an artificial joint becomes infected, it may have to be surgically removed. A second implant is usually possible, but only after the infection has completely cleared. Meanwhile, the person must make do without a joint. Without a hip, for instance, you would need a walker, crutches, or a cane to walk, and your other hip would have to do double duty. To prevent such a catastrophe, people with artificial joints usually take antibiotics in any situation in which they risk getting an infection, such as before routine dental work.

Getting Back on Your Feet after TJR

After surgery, you can expect several weeks or more of intensive physical therapy. Also, people with artificial hips and knees usually need a walker, crutches, or a cane to help them get around for up to several months. And they must avoid certain movements that could dislocate their implants. People with artificial hips, for example, must be careful to not cross their legs at the knees or ankles. If an artificial joint does become dislocated, the surgeon may be able to manipulate the implant back into place by hand without reopening the hip. If not, surgery may be necessary again.

When you've fully recovered, you can resume a fairly active lifestyle, if you follow some general guidelines. "We do not advise doing high-impact activities, such as squash, handball, tennis, downhill skiing, running, or jumping," says Dr. Rothman. Those activities, which put undue stress on hips and knees, can loosen artificial joints. Safe forms of aerobic exercise include bicycling or riding a stationary bike, swimming, and walking, says Dr. Rothman.

Is There a New Joint in Your Future?

As miraculous as joint replacement surgery may be, not everyone is a suitable candidate. Factors like your age, weight, overall health—and even your occupation—can determine whether TJR is right for you.

Even if you are a candidate for TJR, you may have to wait to have this surgery. Your surgeon may want you to postpone surgery for any number of reasons—until you lose weight or recuperate from another health problem, perhaps.

Here are some factors your surgeon will consider when deciding whether to recommend TJR for you.

How old are you? Until recently, surgeons advised many patients to postpone joint replacement surgery until they were older, usually 60 or 65. In general, the older you are, the better your chances for a long-lasting artificial joint. Older people usually are less active, so they put less stress on the implant. That leaves many poor souls sitting around in agony, though, waiting until doctors think they're ripe enough for fixing. Now, with longer-lived cementless implants, more people will be able to have artificial joints (at least in the hips) at a younger age.

"An artificial implant has a finite life span," says Dr. Lisse. "If you're 65 and a joint lasts 20 years, you may eventually need another one. If you're 25, on the other hand, you may need two or three more."

Are you overweight? Obesity puts excess stress on artificial hips and knees and is a major cause of loosened implants, says Dr. Marmar. So overweight people are urged to slim down before getting an artificial joint. Otherwise, the artificial joint won't last as long as it should. And if you're considerably overweight and need a hip replacement, the surgeon will have to rummage around through that extra flesh to get to the hip, making the operation more difficult.

What kind of job do you have? People who do heavy labor, such as construction work, also put stress on artificial joints and have problems with implants loosening. If you have a physically demanding job, your doctor may suggest you postpone surgery until you retire or switch to a less active occupation.

Do you have other serious medical problems? If you have respiratory problems or any type of bacterial infection, if you have suffered a recent stroke or heart attack, or if you have certain other ailments, you'll need to wait until you've fully recovered before having surgery.

Are you willing to undergo several weeks of postoperative rehabilitation? If you don't follow your recovery plan, your artificial joint won't work as well or as painlessly as it should. "This is one operation in your life where you're not going to mend passively," warns Rhoda Lichtenstein, a nurse practitioner who counsels TJR patients at the Einstein-Moss Joint Replacement Center. "You're going to work like you've never worked before!"

Do your knees look worse than they feel? "My knees are hideous," wails one woman who has RA. "But I've quickly discovered that my doctor is not about to perform surgery just to improve my appearance." She is right. Most orthopedic surgeons won't perform joint surgery solely to help you look better. Generally, a joint must be painful or poorly functioning to justify the risks and cost of surgery. The problem with operating on joints for cosmetic reasons is that you "may turn an ugly but asymptomatic area into a good-looking but painful one," says Dr. Fox. "Or an ugly *and* painful one," adds Dr. Lisse.

Other Types of Joint Surgery

While joint replacements and arthroscopic surgery are the best known forms of arthritis surgery, many other surgical procedures can be helpful. Here are some other common procedures.

Synovectomy

This procedure removes the synovial membrane (the tissue that lines the joint). The operation can be done arthroscopically or with open joint surgery. In either case, the surgeon can remove the membrane using a tool with rotating blades that cuts and sucks away the tissue, says Dr. Fox. A synovectomy can relieve pain and prevent joint destruction in a badly inflamed joint because the swollen membrane releases destructive enzymes. People with RA are the most likely candidates for the procedure, which is most often done on knees, wrists, ankles, shoulders, and elbows.

One drawback to the operation is that the synovial membrane can grow back after many months, causing pain and swelling to return. In the past, stiffness also was a problem after surgery, because the joint was cut open and the internal tissues became scarred. Now, however, synovectomy can be done with arthroscopic surgery in most joints. With arthroscopy, stiffness is rarely a problem after surgery, and recovery is much faster.

Joint Fusion

This is a radical procedure in which the cartilage that coats the ends of bones is stripped away and the two bone ends are allowed to heal together. A fused joint can no longer bend, but the operation does provide pain relief and stability. The operation is most often done in the ankle, wrist, finger, and vertebrae. Surprisingly, many people with fused ankles can walk very well, although they may need special shoes. And neighboring joints must assume more functions, which can strain them.

Fusion operations are often the treatment of choice for badly damaged wrists and ankles, where joint replacement has not been very successful and other joints can take up the slack. New surgical practices are making advances in ankle and wrist implants, however, so if your surgeon ever suggests a wrist or ankle fusion, ask about the possiblities of having a new joint installed instead.

Arthroplasty

This term refers to rebuilding joints that have been damaged by arthritis. (Joint replacement surgery is one type of arthroplasty.) In some cases, doctors can salvage a joint by stripping off diseased tissue and resurfacing it with new materials. In the elbow, for example, surgeons sometimes remove damaged joint cartilage and replace it with fascia, a type of connective tissue borrowed from elsewhere in the body. The operation takes about 2 hours, and the recuperation time is similar to recovery from TJR. This surgery is often the operation of choice for people with badly damaged elbows. Although artificial elbows are available, these implants have a higher rate of infection and other complications than do artificial hips and knees, says Dr. Marmar.

Osteotomy

This procedure involves cutting a bone, taking out a wedge, then resetting the bone to put it back into proper position. If the cartilage in your knee is damaged, for example, cutting out a wedge can shift your weight to the other, undamaged side of the knee. Eventually, though, the "good" side will wear out, so essentially this procedure buys you time. It's often used for younger people with arthritis.

Similarly, an osteotomy can correct a deformity of the spine in people with ankylosing spondylitis by putting a bone back into its natural alignment. But it won't relieve pain, because ankylosing spondylitis is a bodywide disease.

A Wait-and-See Approach to Surgery

Needless to say, the decision to have any type of joint surgery is a big one. Fortunately, arthritis surgery is seldom urgent. Most people can take their time deciding whether to have an operation. In fact, waiting sometimes has advantages. Because joint surgery is a rapidly advancing field, surgeons may offer you better options next year than today.

Usually, doctors don't recommend surgery until you've first tried more conservative treatments for your arthritis, such as drugs and physical therapy. If medical treatment helps your condition, or if the disease goes away by itself (as sometimes happens with RA), there's no need to resort to surgery. "As a rule, surgery is considered only after all other methods of treatment have failed," says Dr. Sculco.

Some doctors say you should give nonsurgical treatment for a joint problem at least six months to work before considering surgery. Then, if you continue to have persistent pain despite medical care, ask your doctor to consider referring you to an orthopedic surgeon, suggests Dr. Marmar. Dr. Lisse adds that the need for surgery varies tremendously and depends on the patient and his or her individual condition. Thus, it's sometimes hard to say who needs surgery and who doesn't. If you don't, the surgeon may recommend other treatments, suggest another specialist, or just decide to follow your condition and reevaluate your need for surgery a few months—or a few years—down the road.

Should you indeed need surgery, there's much you can do beforehand to increase your chances for a successful outcome. Here

A Quiz for Your Surgeon

Facing surgery? Don't be afraid to ask questions. This may be your surgeon's 1,200th total hip replacement, but it's your first.

Although your surgeon may not have time to answer every question, a staff nurse often can. Also, ask if information pamphlets or a videotape about your operation are available to educate you about your surgery.

Here's a sampling of questions to ask your doctor before surgery.

1. *What are the risks of this surgery? How likely are these complications?*

Even minor operations can have serious complications, and you have to accept these risks. Also, ask your surgeon to explain the symptoms of postsurgical complications, such as joint infection, so if a problem arises, you'll recognize it and seek prompt medical attention.

2. *Do I have any medical condition that might complicate the surgery or my recovery?*

3. *How do I contact you if I have any problems after surgery?*

Make sure you know what to do if an emergency arises on a weekend or evening or when your surgeon is out of town.

4. *How much pain relief will surgery bring?*

Will the pain relief be permanent, or might the pain return at some point? Find out how much pain the surgery itself will cause and how pain will be treated. Ask how long you will need pain medication to get through the day or night. Also, ask if surgery to correct one joint problem might also relieve pain in neighboring joints.

are some suggestions from doctors interviewed for this book.

Choose an orthopedic surgeon who frequently does the type of operation you're considering. You're more likely to have successful surgery if the surgeon does your particular operation once a week on the average, rather than once a year.

5. *How well will I be able to function after surgery?*

If you need to take a medical leave from work, give up a sport, or otherwise adjust your lifestyle after surgery, it's important to know beforehand. So ask if surgery will have any affect on your love life, work, or hobbies.

6. *Will I need to use crutches, a cane, or a walker after surgery and if so, for how long?*

Also, find out if you will need self-help devices to protect operated joints after surgery.

7. *Will I need physical therapy and if so, for how many sessions a week and where will it be done?*

If you can't drive or arrange transportation, can a therapist come to your home?

8. *Will I need help caring for myself at home after surgery?*

Will you need nursing or other part-time care? Or will a family member suffice?

9. *Are there any preoperative instructions?*

Your doctor may want you to do some specific exercises, lose weight, or change your medications before surgery. For example, many people are told to stop taking aspirin for a week or more before surgery. Aspirin prevents the blood from clotting and could cause unchecked bleeding during or after surgery. If you're taking prednisone, that will also have to be taken into consideration, so mention it to your doctor.

Also, find a surgeon with whom you communicate well. If the surgeon doesn't have time to answer all your questions, make sure there's a staff nurse who can, or find another surgeon.

Look at your X rays. If you've had X rays of your joints, ask the surgeon to show them to you and to point out just what has happened to your joints or bones. (X rays are useful for seeing bones, but not cartilage, muscles, and blood vessels, so they may not always be able to tell your doctor what's going on.)

Get a second opinion. If you're not sure about having surgery, another surgeon's opinion will help to sort out the pros and cons so you can make a sound decision. Even if you're certain surgery is the right option, it's a good idea to confirm your decision and expectations with a second expert. Your original surgeon can suggest a qualified surgeon for a second opinion, but it's a good idea to seek out the second doctor on your own.

Find out all you can about your operation. Ask the surgeon to explain in detail just what he or she plans to do. What benefits can you expect from surgery? What will the recovery process involve? (For other suggestions, see "A Quiz for Your Surgeon" on page 280.)

Ask how many joint procedures are performed each year at the hospital your doctor uses. The more joint surgery they do, the more likely they are to have the latest operating room equipment and a full support staff of specially trained nurses, therapists, and other personnel. If you plan to have joint replacement surgery, for example, look for an institution that does 100 or more of these operations annually, suggests Dr. Sculco.

Get in shape. To speed healing after surgery, your new or repaired joints are going to need the support of strong muscles. "The stronger you start out, the less time your rehabilitation will take," says Martha D. Becker, a physical therapist at the Center for Arthritis and Back Pain in Philadelphia. That doesn't mean you need to be out jogging every morning on a bum knee or hip. But a gentle exercise program to improve strength and flexibility may help. Ask your surgeon to recommend some exercises or possibly refer you to a physical therapist who can design a preoperative exercise program.

Slim down if you're overweight. "With any orthopedic procedure, one of the first things we do is try get the person's body weight down," says Dr. Sculco. Losing weight is most important for surgery on weight-bearing joints, such as hips and knees. Excess weight puts stress on repaired joints, slowing the recovery process. Weight loss is especially important for people having new joints installed.

If you smoke, try to stop, or at least cut down.   If you're looking for a compelling reason to stop smoking, surgery is it. Smokers are more likely than nonsmokers to have problems with general anesthesia, such as an increased risk of developing pneumonia after surgery. And smokers generally have less endurance for the aggressive physical therapy that often follows orthopedic surgery, says Dr. Marmar.

Consider donating your own blood before surgery for use should you need a blood transfusion during your operation.   Using your own blood eliminates any risk of catching blood-borne infections such as AIDS or hepatitis or experiencing an adverse reaction to someone else's blood. "You never want to have to use anybody else's blood if you can help it," says Dr. Sculco. "Your blood is the best blood in the world for you."

Ask about your anesthesia options.   If you need a hip or knee replacement and are a poor candidate for general anesthesia, ask your doctor if you can have the operation with epidural anesthesia, which numbs only the lower part of the body. Although general anesthesia is commonly used for hip and knee replacements, these operations can be done with epidural anesthesia, says Dr. Sculco. In fact, Dr. Sculco prefers to give epidural anesthesia and says this method is used for virtually all hip and knee replacement surgery at his hospital. Similarly, while arthroscopic surgery is usually done with general anesthesia, it too can be done with epidural anesthesia and in some cases, local anesthesia.

Make a strong commitment to surgery and be willing to follow a strict treatment plan after the operation.   The amount of work you put into your rehabiliation program can make the difference between success and failure. If you aren't motivated to follow all your doctor's recommendations to the letter, you're probably not a good candidate for surgery.

Tips for a Speedy Recovery

Should you and your doctor conclude that you could benefit from joint surgery, the operation is just the beginning.

"With every surgical procedure, the surgeon does only half the job," says Bill Warren. "The other 50 percent of the job is up to you." He is right. While the surgeon is in charge of the operation,

What to Take to the Hospital

Going into the hospital for more than a day or two? A few personal items and clothes of your own can help make an extended stay—say, for joint replacement surgery—more comfortable. Consider taking:

• Personal toiletries, including disposable premoistened towels for "spot washing" when you can't shower or bathe.

• A list of the medications you currently take, including the name of the drug, the dosage, and how often you take it.

• Comfortable low-heeled shoes with good support (like aerobic shoes), suitable for walking and physical therapy.

• A set of comfortable, loose clothes for physical therapy, such as a cotton sweat suit. Take clothing that's easy to slip on and off, such as pants with an elastic waistband.

• A bathrobe or housecoat with a zipper (so you won't have to button or pull it on over your head). Avoid floor-length robes—you might trip on the hem.

• A few dollars to pay for television, vending machine snacks, or sundries. Leave your valuables, including your purse, wallet, rings and other jewelry, at home.

• Magazines, a book, stationery, or items to help you pass the time.

the postoperative rehabilitation is equally important, and its effectiveness depends on your efforts. Here are some suggestions for a successful recovery.

Follow your surgeon's rehabilitation plan.   Stick with your physical therapy, if it's recommended. If the exercises start to get boring after a few weeks, listen to some music during exercise or set up a plan to reward yourself for following the therapy.

Be patient.   That advice comes from Howard MacDonald, who's fully recovered from an artificial hip operation. "Don't try to be a hero and overexert yourself. Nature has its own timetable for healing." In the case of major joint surgery, complete recovery may take six months to a year. As you improve, check with your surgeon about when to add new activities, such as golfing or bowling.

Ask a family member or friend to help you rearrange your household for a easier recovery. If you're using crutches or a walker, for example, stow away any scatter rugs to avoid tripping. If you have recently had a hip implant, prevent straining your artificial joints when sitting and rising by using raised toilets and firm chairs. Your knees should be level with or lower than your hips when seated. An occupational therapist can fill you in on exactly what you need at home. (Other precautions are discussed in chapter 12, "Arthritis and Your Love Life," and chapter 13, "Everyday Coping Tips.")

Enlist outside help. Talk to a social worker about any services you may need during your recovery, such as home nursing care or a part-time aide to help with light housework or bathing. A social worker also can tell you if you're eligible for community services, such as Meals-on-Wheels or door-to-door van rides. (Ask to speak to a social worker at the hospital where you have your surgery.)

Be alert to possible complications from surgery. It's important to recognize the signs of complications and to contact your surgeon promptly if you notice anything wrong. In general, you should notify your surgeon right away if you notice any of the following symptoms.

- Increasing pain or swelling in the operated joint or oozing or a change in color or odor in the surgical wound. (These are possible signs of a joint infection or internal bleeding into the wound.)
- Fever over 100°F.
- If you have an artificial joint, signs of infections elsewhere in your body, especially skin lesions or boils, bacterial pneumonia, and urinary tract infections, the symptoms of which include painful, frequent urination or foul-smelling urine. (Also, before you have any dental work, discuss the risks of possible infection with both your doctor and your dentist.)
- Pain, swelling, or loss of function in a body part other than the operated joint. (These are possible signs of a blood clot.)
- Shortness of breath, weakness, or chest pain. (Treat these symptoms as an emergency and call an ambulance, because they could be signs of a blood clot in the lung.)

Ten Ways to Improve
Your Hospital Stay

You say doing time in a hospital isn't your idea of fun? You say your worst nightmare is parading around in a flimsy hospital gown with your posterior on display, while a strange doctor wraps so many bandages around your surgical incision you're later mistaken for the Abominable Snowman?

Cheer up. Although a hospital stay may not compare to a week's vacation in Martinique, it's no jail sentence, either.

If you're having arthroscopic surgery, you probably won't be in the hospital or surgical center for more than a few hours, although an occasional arthroscopy patient requires a one- or two-night hospital stay. If you're having joint replacement surgery, you should prepare for a longer hospital stay, about two weeks for most knee or hip replacements. With a little planning and ingenuity, you can make your visit as pleasant and productive as possible. Here are ten suggestions to help you improve your hospital stay.

• If you have pain after surgery, don't suffer in silence. Ask your nurse for pain medicine the minute you start to feel discomfort, advises Rhoda Lichtenstein, a nurse practitioner at the Einstein-Moss Joint Replacement Center in Philadelphia. "Don't wait until the pain becomes unbearable and you're almost in tears," she says.

• If you expect to have physical therapy while in the hospital, ask your nurse if you can take your pain medicine about an hour before the scheduled session. That way, you will feel less discomfort during exercise, and you'll have a more productive workout.

• Other pain-relief tips: Ask your nurse if you can have a cold pack applied to a painful area. Keeping a limb elevated above the level of the heart also relieves pain by reducing swelling.

• Ask about treatment with a TENS unit, a device that uses a mild

Make no mistake about it: Joint surgery is serious business—nothing to be entered into lightly. But for thousands of people like Betty Warner, Bill Warren, and Howard MacDonald, joint surgery electric current to numb pain. (See chapter 10, "The Three Rs: Relaxation, Rest, and Relief," for more information about TENS.)

• If you're having trouble relaxing or falling asleep, ask your nurse for a back rub or massage. A nurse also can teach you relaxation techniques, such as deep-breathing exercises.

• To pass the time, bring a good novel to read, some magazines with interesting articles, or perhaps crossword puzzles or crewel work.

• Get acquainted with other patients. Most hospitals have a solarium or lounge where patients can get together to chat. "It's uplifting to meet some of the other patients," says Howard MacDonald. MacDonald stayed in the hospital for two weeks after his hip replacement surgery, and he particularly remembers his visits with a charming 90-year-old man.

• Make plans for new activities that will be possible because of your surgery. Perhaps you'll be able to take a trip you've been putting off because you couldn't walk well before surgery. You might bring some travel information and plan where you'd like to go.

• Ask your family to send you a care package with your favorite comfort food, perhaps some home-baked oatmeal cookies or fresh strawberries. (But be sure the food is allowed, if your doctor has put you on a special diet.)

• Tap the expertise of the hospital's support staff. Your nurse and other professionals can share coping tips that will be useful long after you've left the hospital. You might ask your physical therapist how to start a cycling or swimming program, for example. Or ask an occupational therapist for advice on easier ways to do kitchen or yard chores.

makes the difference between enduring pain and immobility and living a full, pain-free life.

CHAPTER

18

Frontiers
in Arthritis Research

The year is 2034—the hundredth anniversary of the American Rheumatism Association. A number of common forms of arthritis are now medical rarities. Rheumatoid arthritis (RA) and lupus have virtually disappeared. (Vaccines prevent both.) Doctors use simple tests to screen the public and determine who is at risk for different types of arthritis. They recommend lifestyle changes to prevent many common forms of arthritis. And people who develop osteoarthritis take pills that stimulate new cartilage growth, reversing the disease.

That scenario—or one close to it—is what today's rheumatologists predict. The outlook for preventing or curing many forms of arthritis is extremely promising. "We're on the threshold of revolutionizing the way we treat arthritis," says Robert Gatter, M.D., chief of rheumatology at Abington Memorial Hospital, associate clinical professor of medicine at the University of Pennsylvania School of Medicine, and director of the Center for Arthritis and Back Pain in Philadelphia.

"Some extraordinarily exciting discoveries are on the horizon," agrees James R. Klinenberg, M.D., a professor of medicine at UCLA School of Medicine and vice president of professional services at Cedars-Sinai Medical Center in Los Angeles.

Hope comes from many medical disciplines, including immunology, surgery, and preventive medicine. Effective new treatments are evolving for autoimmune diseases, such as lupus and RA, based on better understanding of the immune system. (In a survey conducted a few years ago, rheumatologists predicted both these diseases would be wiped out sometime in the next 50 years.) Doctors also foresee the day when surgeons will replace arthritic joints with transplanted healthy human joints, taken from a donor bank, in much the same way cornea transplants are done to restore sight. And doctors also predict that diet and exercise will play larger roles in maintaining joint health before trouble begins.

You won't necessarily have to wait half a century to avail yourself of some of these promising treatments, either. Some new arthritis treatments and tools are already available or on the verge of being adopted. Others will take some years to develop.

Have You Had Your Arthritis Shots?

Tuberculosis, smallpox, polio—these are a few of the diseases that vaccines have nearly wiped out in this century. Before long, RA may be added to the list of medical triumphs. "The potential for a vaccine against rheumatoid arthritis exists," says Daniel J. Wallace, M.D., a rheumatologist and clinical assistant professor of medicine at the UCLA School of Medicine in Los Angeles.

His optimism, shared by many rheumatologists, comes from a growing understanding of what goes wrong in RA. Scientists now know that RA is an autoimmune disease—white blood cells that normally defend the body against foreign organisms turn traitor and attack normal, healthy joints. Researchers are focusing on one type of white blood cell—the T-cell—as the most likely turncoat. Next, they need to locate the exact virus that causes this biochemical reversal.

Right now, this investigation is limited to laboratory animals: Researchers *have* developed a vaccine to prevent and treat RA in rats and mice. But the step from understanding what causes RA in rodents to developing that same understanding—and the appropriate vaccine—for humans is a large one. "Only when the cause is discovered are we likely to have a cure," says Dr. Klinenberg.

When will that be? Some researchers say it will come before the end of the century.

Tests May Identify
Would-Be RA Sufferers

Doctors also expect to be able to test people to find out who is at risk for developing the disease. People who develop RA seem to have a certain genetic makeup. Certain genes—referred to as markers—influence white blood cells in certain ways. But as yet, no one knows how these markers make people vulnerable to the disease.

New Ways to Diagnose Joint Problems
Using MRI

People who have arthritis now can look forward to hearing more about new diagnostic tools within the next few years.

A powerful new imaging technique called magnetic resonance imaging (MRI) enables doctors to see what's happening to your joints *without* using X rays. (Conventional X rays use a form of radiation that poses a slight risk of damaging cells.)

The basis for MRI is a powerful magnetic force 7,000 times stronger than the earth's magnetic field. The MRI machine looks something like a giant Thermos bottle resting on its side. You lie on a table that slides into the center of the machine and for a half hour or so, an invisible magnetic field sends signals from your tissues to a computer, which translates those signals into vivid images of the body in cross-sectional planes. Doctors can interpret those images like X rays.

But unlike X rays, which can show only marked contrast between bones and soft tissues, MRI clearly shows all tissues in considerable detail. An MRI of the knee, for example, shows tendons, cartilage, blood vessels, and the joint's lining. What's more, MRI is painless, with no known side effects. (Anyone with a metal implant, such as an artificial knee, orthopedic pins or rods, or a pacemaker, cannot undergo MRI.)

MRI is already being used in some hospitals to help diagnose a number of types of arthritis, including spinal osteoarthritis and inflammatory arthritis in the knee, as well as a number of nonarthritic conditions. And within a few years, MRI may replace both joint arthroscopy done for diagnostic purposes and a common diagnostic test called an arthrogram.

"With MRI, we can see inside the knee much better than with arthroscopy," says Dr. Klinenberg. (Arthroscopy is described in chapter 17, "Are You a Candidate for Surgery?") "And we can do MRI without probing or cutting into the joint. It's already proving to be extraordinarily useful."

In 1984, only a few hundred hospitals nationwide had an MRI device, according to the American Hospital Association. Now, about a thousand units are in use, and more and more hospitals are expected to install MRI machines in the next few years. By 1995, it is predicted that the number of MRIs in use will double.

Using a related technique called magnetic resonance spectroscopy (MRS), doctors will be able to monitor changes in cell chemistry without taking tissue samples or putting probes into the body. In other words, where MRI provides a precise picture of a joint, spectroscopy analyzes tissue changes that can signal the presence of arthritis or other disease. Although MRS is still in its infancy, the technique may one day help your doctor tell in a flash, for example, whether your knee is swollen because you have an infection, RA, or some other problem.

New Breakthroughs in Drug Therapy

A number of promising new arthritis medicines are emerging. Some have just been approved or are on the verge of being approved; others are being developed and tested.

Diclofenac sodium. This new anti-inflammatory drug has been popular for years everywhere but in the United States. It received the Food and Drug Administration's (FDA) stamp of approval in late 1988, so by the time you read this, diclofenac sodium (brand name Voltaren) should be available by prescription for osteoarthritis, RA, and ankylosing spondylitis. It has a particular benefit for older people: It's quickly eliminated from the bloodstream but continues to work in the joint fluid for up to 24 hours. For this reason, it's less likely than some other anti-inflammatories to build up to toxic levels. This drug is not a cure-all, however, and otherwise is no more effective than other nonsteroidal anti-inflammatory drugs (NSAIDs).

Misoprostol. This drug (brand name Cytotec) may safely prevent or heal side effects associated with use of aspirin, even while people continue to take aspirin. Misoprostol is a synthetic version of a prostaglandin, a hormonelike substance that, among other things, seems to protect and heal the stomach lining. And that's important, because if you rely on aspirin to relieve arthritis pain, you may have traded your aching joints for a miserable stomachache. Used regularly, aspirin frequently causes stomach bleeding and ulcers.

As it stands now, if you develop an ulcer, your doctor probably will take you off arthritis drugs until it heals, leaving you with few (or no) medications to ease joint pain and swelling. More seriously, bleeding ulcers can be life-threatening. Gastric bleeding is ultimately fatal in about 10 percent of RA patients who are hospitalized for drug-induced ulcers, according to a report in the medical journal *Patient Care.*

Misoprostol could be a blessing for the estimated 25 percent of arthritis patients who develop aspirin-induced ulcers after long-term therapy.

So far the drug seems to be safe and effective. In one study, rheumatologist Sanford Roth, M.D., and his colleagues examined 239 arthritis patients who already had ulcers or some gastrointestinal bleeding due to aspirin. While maintaining their aspirin dose, the patients were given either misoprostol or a placebo (a look-alike, fake pill). Within two months, stomach problems had disappeared in 78 percent of the misoprostol patients, compared to 29 percent of those in the placebo group.

This stomach-saving tablet also may be used with common NSAIDs, such as Feldene, Clinoril, and Motrin.

Like all drugs, misoprostol does have some side effects (like diarrhea). But these symptoms are usually mild and go away in time, says Robert Bell, M.D., associate director of medical and scientific information for G. D. Searle and Company, the drug company that makes misoprostol. (Because prostaglandins can cause uterine contractions, there is some question about whether the drug should be used by fertile women of childbearing age.)

Misoprostol was approved by the FDA in February, 1989, and is now available in the U.S. Previously, it had been approved as an anti-ulcer drug in 43 other countries. (*Editor's Note:* In France, this drug is sold under the name RU 486 and is sometimes used to abort unwanted pregnancies. Our discussion of misoprostol is limited to its use in conjunction with arthritis and ulcers.)

If you have arthritis and are interested in misoprostol, check with your family physician or rheumatologist about its availability and whether you would benefit from taking this medicine.

Therfectin. This new drug is actually a carbohydrate—amprilose—and it may take the starch out of arthritis. The drug seems to alter the immune system, preventing damage to joints, according to Jacques R. Caldwell, M.D., of the University of Florida College of Medicine in Gainesville. About 70 percent of patients treated with the drug have had a decrease in swelling, joint tenderness, and the number of joints involved. And studies seem to indicate that it has fewer, milder side effects than other drugs. Therfectin is currently in clinical trials.

Interferon. This older drug may make a comeback. In the 1970s, interferon was hailed as the up-and-coming miracle cure for everything from the common cold to cancer. Well, interferon is still around, even though it hasn't lived up to initial expectations. One form of the drug, gamma interferon, may be useful in the treatment of RA.

Gamma interferon is a hormonelike substance that regulates immune processes. Preliminary evidence shows that injections of gamma interferon ease joint swelling and pain in some people with RA. If doctors can figure out *how* it helps RA, they may be able to work backward and figure out *why* it works. "It's a completely new type of therapy," says Grant Cannon, M.D., a rheumatologist at the University of Utah Medical Center in Salt Lake City, who has conducted studies of how people with RA respond to interferon.

Doctors say gamma interferon will not be available as a prescription drug until they can prove it's safe and effective, which will take at least several years. At this point, gamma interferon doesn't work any better than drugs now in use. Also, it causes some disturbing side effects, including fever and flulike symptoms.

Cyclosporine. This drug, principally used to prevent rejection of organ transplants, may be useful for easing symptoms of RA. In preliminary studies, the drug was shown to reduce joint pain, swelling, and stiffness in people with severe arthritis. But for now, the jury is still out on its value as an arthritis drug. Cyclosporine can cause serious side effects, including kidney damage, high blood pressure, and stomach upset.

Nerve blockers. These drugs provide a new approach to treating RA. Rather than trying to bolster a faulty immune system, they work on the nervous system. "I think the role of the nervous system in arthritis is very powerful," says Jon Levine, M.D., Ph.D., an assistant professor of medicine at the University of California in San Francisco. If he's right, it could open up a whole new spectrum of treatments for RA (and quite possibly for other types of arthritis as well).

Dr. Levine theorizes that nerve endings in the joints contribute to arthritis pain and swelling. His idea provides a neat explanation for some puzzling observations. Doctors have long known, for example, that stroke patients who have lost some function on one side of the body rarely develop arthritis on that side. On their normal side, however, full-blown arthritis can develop. This relationship is true for RA, as well as for gout and osteoarthritis.

Two types of nerves in joints are the focus of Dr. Levine and his colleagues. The first are sensory fibers that carry pain messages from the joints to the brain. These nerve endings are filled with a chemical messenger called substance P. When substance P is released into the joints of rats, it causes inflammation. The higher the level of substance P in the joints of rats the more severe the arthritis.

Dr. Levine is also investigating the sympathetic nervous system, the part of the nervous system that speeds up your heart rate and automatically prepares your body to fight or flee in a taxing situation. Sympathetic nerve endings control a number of different joint functions. Destroying part of the nervous system in rats makes it much harder to induce arthritis in the animals, which suggests that these nerves, too, contribute to pain and swelling.

Dr. Levine's theory might also explain why stress—which involves the nervous system—so often triggers arthritic flare-ups.

In a preliminary study in people, Dr. Levine and his team tested a drug called guanethidine, which blocks the sympathetic nervous system. When the drug was intravenously infused into the arms of some patients, elbow, wrist, and hand pain decreased and hand strength increased. (During the drug infusion, the patients wore tight blood pressure cuffs around their arms, which prevented guanethidine from circulating to other parts of the body and causing unwanted side effects.) Although it is impractical to use guanethidine as a standard arthritis drug, the researchers hope to find other, more specific drugs that will block the harmful effects of sympathetic nerves on joints.

Better Treatments for Osteoarthritis

Preliminary evidence shows promise for still other intriguing arthritis treatments. While it's too soon to talk about curing osteoarthritis, doctors do foresee exciting new treatments ahead for humankind's oldest and most common disease.

One of the most promising areas of research addresses the factors that control cartilage growth. (In osteoarthritis, you'll recall, the firm, rubbery cartilage that covers your bones becomes pitted and frayed and in time may wear away completely. Without their protective coating, bones that form joints grate on each other, making movement painful.) Doctors hope to find drugs that stimulate cartilage growth and repair, reversing joint destruction.

"At the moment, the results are promising, because we're learning what's responsible for cartilage regeneration," says Dr. Klinenberg.

One current development that may help protect cartilage is the drug S-adenosylmethionine (SAMe). It works like aspirin to reduce joint pain and swelling. (It may also help prevent ulcers.) But it *also* promotes the manufacture of key structural molecules in cartilage. What's more, SAMe prevents a form of experimentally induced osteoarthritis in rabbits. But no one has shown that SAMe prevents arthritis in people, and the drug may be just a forerunner of more powerful drugs to come. (SAMe has been widely tested in Europe, but at this writing, it isn't available as a prescription drug in the United States.)

While some researchers are figuring out how to grow more cartilage, others are working to stop unwanted bone growth. As the cartilage wears away, the bone goes on a growing spree, as if to compensate for the cartilage loss. Painful bony spurs, or osteophytes, often grow around the joints. Learning how to control this unruly bone growth is just as important as revving up the cartilage, says John Bland, M.D., a rheumatologist and osteoarthritis researcher at the University of Vermont College of Medicine in Burlington. He predicts that in the future, naturally produced hormones called bone-growth factors will be used to prevent osteophytes and make the bones behave.

Radiation Synovectomy:
Knee Surgery without the Scalpel

Having a radioactive element, or radioisotope, injected into your knee sounds like a strange and scary method of treating RA. But this new technique can temporarily ease knee pain and swelling and help people walk better, say surgeons who developed the procedure.

In RA, the lining inside the joint cavity (the synovium) sometimes grows out of control, causing pain and swelling and releasing harmful enzymes that may eventually destroy the joint. To suppress this wayward growth of tissue, doctors first try to treat the problem with drugs. If this is unsuccessful, the doctor may recommend a synovectomy, a surgical procedure to remove the diseased joint lining.

But a few years ago, some surgeons wondered why people should go through the ordeal of joint surgery when a single injection might do the same job. They figured out a way to inject the knee with a radioisotope that clobbered the synovium without leaking out of the joint to damage other tissues. The technique, developed in England and refined by Clement B. Sledge, M.D., an orthopedic surgeon at Harvard Medical School, so far has shown promising results. In one study, 84 percent of a group of patients who had their knees injected with radioactive material (in this case, something called dysprosium 165-ferric hydroxide macro-aggregate) continued to have reduced pain and swelling a year later. (Dr. Sledge and his colleagues perform the procedure on a regular basis at the Brigham and Women's Hospital, Boston.)

The procedure is considered safe because it destroys the diseased synovium without harming healthy tissues, explains David R. Lionberger, M.D., an orthopedic surgeon and assistant clinical instructor at Baylor College of Medicine in Houston. (He worked with Dr. Sledge to develop the technique and now performs about 25 radiation synovectomies each year.) Only a minuscule amount of radiation escapes into the circulatory system, and it decays so quickly that almost all of it is gone within a day.

"Many people with arthritis want an alternative to surgery," says Dr. Lionberger. "And there's no reason to have surgery if an injection will do the same thing."

The new procedure has many advantages over its surgical counterpart, claims Dr. Lionberger. Unlike surgery, which may involve a hospital stay, radiation synovectomy can be done as an outpatient procedure. Patients need only a local anesthetic to numb the injection site, and most go home the same day.

Surgery usually involves lengthy rehabilitation, poses the risk of bleeding or infection, and leaves the joint stiff afterward—all of which are results of cutting into muscles and joint tissues. Radiation synovectomy, in contrast, avoids those complications and doesn't limit the knee's range of motion, says Dr. Lionberger.

But the new procedure has its drawbacks, too. The joint lining can grow back in time, instigating pain and swelling once again. If that happens, the joint can be reinjected periodically. More critically, surgeons don't yet know if the radiation will have long-term side effects. Leaking radiation, however minute the amount, could cause cancer in healthy cells—a major concern. Still, Dr. Lionberger is optimistic about the technique and predicts that in the next few years doctors will use the procedure to treat other joints, most likely the shoulder, wrist, and hip.

With so many intriguing possibilities on the horizon, it's possible that medical research will revolutionize arthritis treatment within a decade or two.

Index

Page references in *italic* indicate tables.